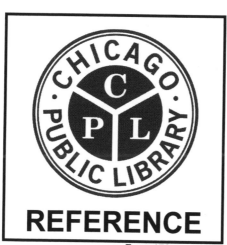

American Public Health Association
VITAL AND HEALTH STATISTICS MONOGRAPHS

THE FREQUENCY OF THE RHEUMATIC DISEASES

THE FREQUENCY OF THE RHEUMATIC DISEASES

SIDNEY COBB

1971 / HARVARD UNIVERSITY PRESS
Cambridge, Massachusetts

Distributed in Great Britain by Oxford University Press, London
This material has been copyrighted to insure its accurate quotation and use.
Permission to reprint may be granted upon presentation of an adequate statement concerning the material to be used and the manner of its incorporation in
other texts.

Library of Congress Catalog Card Number 72-158427
SBN 674-32325-4
Printed in the United States of America

DEDICATION

To my father who suffered with rheumatoid disease and to my
mother who made it possible for him to carry on an enormously
productive career despite his illness and disability.

PREFACE

This book concerns a relatively new subject. Very few references will be found to survey work done before the middle of the present century. Although there were a few pioneers who gathered statistics about rheumatism in the 1920's, it was not until the early 1950's that serious, continuing work on the epidemiology of the rheumatic diseases was undertaken both in England and in the United States. Since that time the field has progressed from simple prevalence surveys through methodologic developments to epidemiologic investigations of etiologic factors. It is reasonable to expect that progress will be even more rapid in the decade to come.

My attempt has been to write an interpretive book. The approach has been to put the information together in what seemed to me the most useful way, which is quite different from simple cataloging of the literature. Many of the tables are new juxtapositions of old data; some are worthy of study in their own right, for they suggest ideas beyond those they were designed to bring out. If this book stimulates further research, the effort involved in its preparation will be fully rewarded.

I have tried to express my opinions in the first person. If my biases are reflected in the selection of data to be presented or in possible distortions of original reports, I can only hope that the corrective of time will purge my sins.

It would be quite impossible to identify all those who have indirectly contributed to this monograph, but the following cannot go unrecognized. It was John Everett Gordon who started me on what has turned out to be eighteen years of research on the epidemiology of rheumatic disease. Thomas A. Burch was to have been a coauthor; although the press of other duties prevented him from full participation, his contributions in the early stages were substantial. Mortimer Spiegelman was supportive and patient in his role as coordinator of this monograph series. His death was a great loss to all of us who worked with him and valued his friendship.

George Brooks has been a long-time associate on the laboratory side of the research and contributed especially to the sections dealing with the rheumatoid factor. Alphonse T. Masi, John S. Lawrence, Ivan Duff, and Horace J. Dodge have contributed by thoughtful reading of the manuscript. Special thanks go to Edith Chen, Suzanne Dressler, Theresa D'Arms, Gail Kohn, and Barbara Betsey who in turn assisted me with the literature search and helped to keep the files in order. Judith Baughn has rendered invaluable service in typing the manuscript and attending to the many details associated with the completion of such a task. Finally, I am particularly grateful to my wife, Rosalind, for her patience and support.

I am indebted to the National Center for Health Statistics for mortality and morbidity data. These data are referenced without date or notation in the bibliography. I am grateful to the following for permission to republish certain figures:

Figures 3.1 and 3.2 are reprinted with permission from the *Journal of Occupational Medicine*, vol. 5, no. 1 (1963), pp. 10–16. Copyright by the Industrial Medical Association.

Figure 3.3 is reprinted with permission from the *American Journal of Public Health*, vol. 52, no. 7 (1962), pp. 1119–1125. Copyright by the American Public Health Association.

Figure 5.2 is reprinted with permission of the publisher and Dr. J. S. Lawrence from *The Epidemiology of Chronic Rheumatism*, J. H. Kellgren, M. R. Jeffrey, and John Ball, eds. (Oxford: Blackwell Scientific Publications, 1963) vol. 1, p. 99.

Figure 6.1 is reprinted with permission of the publisher and Dr. William M. Mikkelsen from the *American Journal of Medicine*, vol. 39 (1964), p. 244.

Quotations of diagnostic criteria are reprinted with permission from the *Bulletin on the Rheumatic Diseases*, vol. 17 (1967), pp. 453–458. Copyright by the Arthritis Foundation.

The research herein reported has been supported by the following grants from the United States Public Health Service: A–308, A–1607, AM–06928, KO5–MH16709, HS–00572, and CH–00075.

The final editing of the manuscript was accomplished during a sabbatical leave in the Department of Epidemiology, Harvard School of Public Health. Mimi Jacobs was most helpful in typing the necessary changes.

Ann Arbor   S.C.
December 1969

CONTENTS

Foreword by James R. Kimmey, M.D.   xvii

Notes on Tables and Figures   xxi

1. BASIC CONCEPTS   1

    1.0 Introduction   1
    1.1 Diseases   1
    1.2 Epidemiology   1
    1.3 Painful Swelling of Joints   1
    1.4 The Principle of Severity Gradient   2
    1.5 Remittency   2
    1.6 Pain   4
    1.7 Age-Sex Adjustment   4
    1.8 Etiology   4
    1.9 History   5

2. RHEUMATIC COMPLAINTS   6

    2.0 Introduction   6
    2.1 Sources of Data   6
    2.2 Total Disability   7
    2.3 Partial Disability   8
    2.4 Medical Treatment   9
    2.5 Complaints   11
    2.6 Effects of Age, Sex, and Heavy Work   14
    2.7 Overview   16

3. THE FREQUENCY OF RHEUMATOID DISEASE   17

    3.0 Introduction   17
    3.1 Diagnostic Criteria   18
    3.2 Validity and Reproducibility of the Clinical Criteria   20
    3.3 Validity and Reproducibility of the X-ray Criterion   22
    3.4 Validity and Reproducibility of Serologic Tests   24
    3.5 Interview Approaches   26
    3.6 Relationships   27

3.7 Point Prevalence   28
3.8 Incidence   29
3.9 Patterns of Manifestations over Time   30
3.10 Medical Care and Disability   36
3.11 Mortality   38
3.12 Overview   41

4.   THE EPIDEMIOLOGY OF RHEUMATOID DISEASE   42

4.0 Introduction   42
4.1 Age and Sex   42
4.2 Time and Place   44
4.3 Race   48
4.4 Family Structure   49
4.5 Socioeconomic Status   51
4.6 Season   51
4.7 Heredity   51
4.8 Association with Other Diseases   52
4.9 Infection   53
4.10 Trauma   55
4.11 Social Stress   56
4.12 Personality   57
4.13 Early Life   57
4.14 Affect and Behavior   58
4.15 Negative Association with Psychosis   60
4.16 A Theory   61

5.   DEGENERATIVE JOINT DISEASE   63

5.0 Introduction   63
5.1 Pain   63
5.2 Clinical Syndromes   64
5.3 Observer Variation   66
5.4 Prevalence of Osteoarthrosis   67
5.5 Prevalence of Disk Degeneration   69
5.6 Etiology   70
5.7 Epidemiologic Evidence for the Wear-and-Tear Theory   71
5.8 Heredity   76
5.9 Significance   78
5.10 Overview   79

6. GOUT AND HYPERURICEMIA 81
   6.0 Introduction. The Disease 81
   6.1 Prevalence 82
   6.2 Incidence 84
   6.3 Associations 84
   6.4 Relation of Serum Uric Acid Level to Frequency of
       Gout 85
   6.5 Serum Uric Acid Levels 87
   6.6 Factors Associated with Uric Acid Level 90
   6.7 Factors Precipitating Acute Gout 93
   6.8 Genetics 94
   6.9 Control Measures 95
   6.10 Overview 96

7. THE CONNECTIVE-TISSUE DISORDERS 97

   7.0 Introduction 97
   7.1 The Disorders 97
   7.2 Mortality 97
   7.3 Polyarteritis Nodosa 101
   7.4 Dermtomyositis and Scleroderma 102
   7.5 Lupus Erythematosus 102
   7.6 Overview 104

8. ANKYLOSING SPONDYLITIS AND JUVENILE
   ARTHRITIS 105

   8.0 Introduction 105
   8.1 Ankylosing Spondylitis 105
   8.2 Observer Variation 106
   8.3 Prevalence 107
   8.4 Association with Other Diseases 108
   8.5 Heredity 109
   8.6 Juvenile Rheumatoid Arthritis 110
   8.7 Onset 111
   8.8 Mortality 111
   8.9 Prevalence and Incidence 111
   8.10 Heredity 112
   8.11 Environmental Factors 113
   8.12 Overview 114

9.   CODA   115

9.0 Introduction   115
9.1 Relative Disability and Need for Care   115
9.2 Overview   118
9.3 Directions for the Future   119

BIBLIOGRAPHY   123

INDEX   145

TABLES

2.1 Severity gradient of rheumatism in the United States, 1936   7

2.2 Annual incidence per 1,000 of arthritis disabling for 8 days or more in personnel of the Metropolitan Life Insurance Company for two time periods   8

2.3 Days of disability per 1,000 persons per year due to arthritis and rheumatism as reported in household interviews in the United States, July 1957–June 1959   9

2.4 Medical care for arthritis and related conditions compared to total medical care for Group Health Insurance   10

2.5 The distribution of persons by gradient of arthritis and classification on certain questions about arthritis and rheumatism, lifetime prevalence rates per 1,000 persons 15 years of age and over for the Arsenal Health District of Pittsburgh, 1952 to 1954   11

2.6 The frequency of medically verified rheumatic complaints in three surveys in the United States compared with studies in other countries   13

2.7 Number of persons per 1,000 with various degrees of severity of arthritis and rheumatism as reported in household interview by sex, with sex ratios   16

3.1 Agreement between observers as percent of total reported positive by either observer at independent examinations   21

3.2 The diagnostic value for rheumatoid arthritis of X-ray, serology and interview techniques. Selected data from population samples   23

3.3 The relationship between the more common tests[a] for rheumatoid factor in population samples; percent of those positive on either test who are positive on both tests   25

3.4 The relationship among the findings in two major surveys   27

3.5 Age-sex adjusted* rates per 100 persons age 35–64 for probable plus definite rheumatoid arthritis by A.R.A. criteria, from selected large studies   29

3.6 The apparent progression of rheumatoid arthritis as observed in a group of 331 employed men over a 28-month period   32

3.7 The proportion of men meeting the diagnostic criteria for probable rheumatoid arthritis by the end of the fourth month and by the end of the twenty-eighth month given the specified observations during the first four months of the observation period   37

3.8 Number of consultations and number of patients consulting for rheumatoid arthritis per 1,000 persons per year for selected general practices in England and Wales, 1955   40

4.1 The frequency per 100 persons of various degrees of severity of rheumatoid arthritis and of certain manifestations of the disease by sex, with sex ratios   44

4.2 The point prevalence of rheumatoid arthritis (A.R.A. probable plus definite) in various surveys, rates per 100 persons of specified age and sex   46

4.3 The point prevalence of rheumatoid arthritis (A.R.A. probable and

definite) per 100 United States residents age 35–64 by race, age
adjusted to the U.S. population of 1940   48

4.4   Point prevalence rates per 100 persons for rheumatoid arthritis in
       United States residents aged 35–64 by sex, race and place of resi-
       dence, age adjusted to the U.S. population of 1940   50

4.5   The relationship between rheumatoid arthritis and the reporting of
       mother as arbitrary and resented   58

4.6   The relation of anger impulsiveness to rheumatoid arthritis in three
       separate studies   59

5.1   Correlation between and within observers in the assessment of osteo-
       arthrosis in various joints and groups of joints   66

5.2   The prevalence per 100 persons X-rayed of disk degeneration in the
       cervical, dorsal and lumbar spines of males and females from Leigh
       and Wensleydale, England   70

5.3   Percent of persons with the indicated degree of anatomical evidence
       of osteoarthrosis, data on 1,002 cadavers   72

5.4   The relation of obesity to osteoarthrosis in males and females
       combined   73

5.5   The relative frequency of male admissions to the Royal Mineral
       Water Hospital in Bath, England, for osteoarthritis by type of work 74

5.6   Standardized morbidity ratios for osteoarthritis and displacement of
       intervertebral disk for selected light and heavy occupations among
       persons receiving United States social security benefits for disability 76

6.1   Prevalence of gouty persons by sex in various populations   83

6.2   Prevalence of persons with gout by serum uric acid level at age 40
       and over, by sex, in Framingham, Massachusetts, and Tecumseh,
       Michigan   86

6.3   The probability of having gout or renal lithiasis before age 54 by the
       maximum of six serum uric acid determinations in the last 10 years,
       Framingham, Massachusetts   87

6.4   Mean serum uric acid levels as determined by the spectrophotometric
       uricase method for certain Caucasian populations   88

6.5   Relationship between serum uric acid level and ratio of body weight
       to ideal weight at age 25 for 134 blue collar employees at a metal
       refining plant   91

6.6   Prevalence of persons with gout among the relatives of persons with
       gout   94

7.1   Mortality rates by age and sex for selected rheumatic diseases, United
       States, 1959–1961   99

7.2   Adjusted mortality rates by sex and color, marital status, and geo-
       graphic region for selected rheumatic diseases, United States, 1959–
       1961   100

8.1   Observer variation among three physicians reading X-rays of the
       sacroiliac joints for evidence of ankylosing spondylitis   106

8.2   The frequency of agreed-upon sacroiliac (S-I) changes indicative of
       ankylosing spondylitis in seven male populations by age, changes of
       grade 2–4 according to the *Atlas of Standard Radiographs* based on
       A–P films of the pelvis read by three observers   108

8.3 The prevalence per 100 persons of ankylosing spondylitis among
     relatives of patients with that disease by degree of relatedness   110
9.1 Disability due to arthritis and rheumatism in Leigh, Lancashire,
     England, by diagnosis   116
9.2 Consultation and patient consulting rates per 1,000 population by
     sex and selected diagnoses for 106 practices in England and Wales,
     1955–56   117
9.3 Percent distribution by diagnosis in several severity categories   118

FIGURES

1.1 Illustrative frequency distributions by degree of severity: rabies, diphtheria and measles compared. 3

2.1 The prevalence per 1,000 persons by age of various degrees of severity of rheumatic affliction as reported in household interviews, United States, July 1957 to June 1959, based on 73,000 interviews. (U.S. National Health Survey, 1960*b*.) 15

3.1 Nine cases selected from the Oak Ridge (Tennessee) Arthritis Study to illustrate different symptom patterns over time. At the left margin are the ARA Criteria: M S = morning stiffness; P on M or T = pain on motion or tenderness; OBS SW = observed swelling; SW 2+JTS = swelling observed in two or more joints; SYM SW = symmetrical swelling. The superscripts P and D refer to the times at which diagnoses of probable or definite rheumatoid arthritis were made. Shading indicates that particular manifestation was present at that monthly screening. The heavy line at the bottom of each case is interrupted if that man was not screened in that month. (Reproduced with permission from Lincoln and Cobb, 1963.) 31

3.2 Cumulated frequency of persons diagnosed rheumatoid arthritis, Oak Ridge (Tennessee), September 1957 through December 1960. (Reproduced with permission from Lincoln and Cobb, 1963.) 34

3.3 Frequency distribution of men according to the proportion of time spent with observable evidence of pain on motion or tenderness in their joints. Men under 45 compared with men 45 and over. (Reproduced with permission from Cobb, 1962.) 35

3.4 Days of sickness attributed to rheumatoid arthritis per 1,000 insured persons per year. (Ministry of Health of Great Britain, 1924.) 39

4.1 Prevalence of probable rheumatoid arthritis in the continental United States by age. (National Center for Health Statistics, 1966*b*.) 43

4.2 Schematic presentation of epidemiologically derived hypotheses about the etiology of rheumatoid arthritis. The black box remains the province of clinical investigation. 62

5.1 Radiological osteoarthrosis of the hands, grades 2 to 4, by age, for three populations. (Burch, 1967; National Center for Health Statistics, 1966*a*; Blumberg *et al.*, 1961.) 68

5.2 Prevalence of grade 2 to 4 degenerative change in individual disks in random samples of 100 males and 100 females aged 35 and over. Males: black; females: stippled. (Reproduced with permission from Lawrence *et al.*, 1963.) 69

6.1 Serum uric acid levels by age and sex. Tecumseh, Michigan, 1959 to 1960. (Reproduced with permission from Mikkelsen *et al.*, 1965.) 90

8.1 Distribution of onsets among hospital cases of juvenile rheumatoid arthritis by age and sex, three-year moving averages calculated from Ansell and Bywaters (1963). 112

FOREWORD

Rapid advances in medical and allied sciences, changing patterns in medical care and public health programs, an increasingly health-conscious public, and the rising concern of voluntary agencies and government at all levels in meeting the health needs of the people necessitate constant evaluation of the country's health status. Such an evaluation, which is required not only for an appraisal of the current situation, but also to refine present goals and to gauge our progress toward them, depends largely upon a study of vital and health statistics records.

Opportunity to study mortality in depth emerges when a national census furnishes the requisite population data for the computation of death rates in demographic and geographic detail. Prior to the 1960 census of population there had been no comprehensive analysis of this kind. It therefore seemed appropriate to build up for intensive study a substantial body of death statistics for a three-year period centered around that census year.

A detailed examination of the country's health status must go beyond an examination of mortality statistics. Many conditions such as arthritis, rheumatism, and mental diseases are much more important as causes of morbidity than of mortality. Also, an examination of health status should not be based solely upon current findings, but should take into account trends and whatever pertinent evidence has been assembled through local surveys and from clinical experience.

The proposal for such an evaluation, to consist of a series of monographs, was made to the Statistics Section of the American Public Health Association in October 1958 by Mortimer Spiegelman, and a Committee on Vital and Health Statistics Monographs was authorized, with Mr. Spiegelman as Chairman, a position he held until his death on March 25, 1969. The members of this Committee and of the Editorial Advisory Subcommittee created later are:

Committee on Vital and Health Statistics Monographs

Carl L. Erhardt, D.Sc., Chairman
Paul M. Densen, D.Sc.
Robert D. Grove, Ph.D.
Clyde V. Kiser, Ph.D.
Felix Moore

George Rosen, M.D., Ph.D.
William H. Stewart, M.D.*
Conrad Taeuber, Ph.D.
Paul Webbink
Donald Young, Ph.D.

*Withdrew June 1964

The early history of this undertaking is described in a paper presented at the 1962 Annual Conference of the Milbank Memorial Fund.[1] The Committee on Vital and Health Statistics Monographs selected the topics to be included in the series and also suggested candidates for authorship. The frame of reference was extended by the Committee to include other topics in vital and health statistics than mortality and morbidity, namely fertility, marriage, and divorce. Conferences were held with authors to establish general guidelines for the preparation of the manuscripts.

Support for this undertaking in its preliminary stages was received from the Rockefeller Foundation, the Milbank Memorial Fund, and the Health Information Foundation. Major support for the required tabulations, for writing and editorial work, and for the related research of the monograph authors was provided by the United States Public Health Service (Research Grant CH 00075, formerly GM 08262). Acknowledgment should also be made to the Metropolitan Life Insurance Company for the facilities and time that were made available to Mr. Spiegelman before his retirement in December 1966, after which he devoted his major time to administer the undertaking and to serve as general editor. Without his abiding concern over each monograph in the series and his close work with the authors, the completion of the series might have been in grave doubt. The published volumes will be a fitting memorial to Mr. Spiegelman even though his name does not appear as an author.

The New York City Department of Health allowed Dr. Carl L. Erhardt to allocate part of his time to administrative details for the series from April to December 1969, when he retired to assume a more active role. The National Center for Health Statistics, under the

---

[1] Mortimer Spiegelman, "The Organization of the Vital and Health Statistics Monograph Program," *Emerging Techniques in Population Research (Proceedings of the 1962 Annual Conference of the Milbank Memorial Fund*; New York: Milbank Memorial Fund, 1963), p. 230. See also Mortimer Spiegelman, "The Demographic Viewpoint in the Vital and Health Statistics Monographs Project of the American Public Health Association," *Demography*, vol. 3, no. 2 (1966), p. 574.

supervision of Dr. Grove and Miss Alice M. Hetzel, undertook the sizable tasks of planning and carrying out the extensive mortality tabulations for the 1959–1961 period. Dr. Taeuber arranged for the cooperation of the Bureau of the Census at all stages of the project in many ways, principally by furnishing the required population data used in computing death rates and by undertaking a large number of varied special tabulations. As the sponsor of the project, the American Public Health Association furnished assistance through Dr. Thomas R. Hood, its Deputy Executive Director.

Because of the great variety of topics selected for monograph treatment, authors were given an essentially free hand to develop their manuscripts as they desired. Accordingly, the authors of the individual monographs bear the full responsibility for their manuscripts, and their opinions and statements do not necessarily represent the viewpoints of the American Public Health Association or of the agencies with which they may be affiliated.

James R. Kimmey, M.D.
Executive Director
American Public Health Association

NOTES ON TABLES AND FIGURES

1. Regarding 1959–1961 mortality data:
   a. Deaths relate to those occurring in the United States (including Alaska and Hawaii);
   b. Deaths are classified by place of resident (if pertinent);
   c. Fetal deaths are excluded;
   d. Deaths of unknown age, marital status, nativity, or other characteristics have not been distributed into the known categories, but are included in their totals;
   e. Deaths were classified by cause according to the *Seventh Revision of the International Statistical Classification of Diseases, Injuries, and Causes of Death* (Geneva: World Health Organization, 1957);
   f. All death rates are average annual rates per 100,000 population in the category specified, as recorded in the United States census of April 1, 1960;
   g. Age-adjusted rates were computed by the direct method using the age distribution of the total United States population in the census of April 1, 1940 as a standard.[1]
2. Symbols used in tables of data:
   --- Data not available;
   ... Category not applicable;
   - Quantity zero;
   0.0 Quantity more than zero but less than 0.05;
   *Figure does not meet the standard of reliability or precision:
   a) Rate or ratio based on less than 20 deaths;
   b) Percentage or median based on less than 100 deaths;
   c) Age-adjusted rate computed from age-specific rates where more than half of the rates were based on frequencies of less than 20 deaths.
3. Case rates and death rates are annual rates per 100,000 mid-year population in the categories specified.
4. Geographic classification:[2]
   a. Standard Metropolitan Statistical Areas (SMSA's): except in the New England States, "an SMSA is a county or a group of contiguous counties which contains at least one city of 50,000 inhabitants or more or 'twin cities' with a combined population of at least 50,000 in the 1960 census. In addition, contiguous counties are included in an SMSA if, according to specified criteria, they are (a) essentially metropolitan in character and (b) socially and economically integrated with the central city or cities." In New England, the Division of Vital Statistics of the National Center for Health Statistics uses, instead of the definition just cited, Metropolitan State Economic Areas (MSEA's) established by the Bureau of the Census, which are made up of county units.

[1] Mortimer Spiegelman and H. H. Marks, "Empirical Testing of Standards for the Age Adjustment of Death Rates by the Direct Method," *Human Biology*, 38:280 (September 1966).
[2] *Vital Statistics of the United States, 1960* (Washington, D.C.: National Center for Health Statistics, 1963), vol. 2 *(Mortality)*, pt. A, sec. 7, p. 8.

b. Metropolitan and nonmetropolitan: "Counties which are included in SMSA's or, in New England, MSEA's are called metropolitan counties; all other counties are classified as nonmetropolitan."
c. Metropolitan counties may be separated into those containing at least one central city of 50,000 inhabitants or more or twin cities as specified previously, and into metropolitan counties without a central city.

THE FREQUENCY OF THE
RHEUMATIC DISEASES

1 / BASIC CONCEPTS

1.0 Introduction. In order for the reader to understand this monograph, it is important that he be aware of what it is and is not about, and of some of the principles both established and assumed that underlie its development.

1.1 Diseases. The first concern will be with the sum of rheumatic complaints. Then attention will turn to rheumatoid arthritis, osteoarthrosis, and gout in that order. Finally, there will be two chapters on some of the less frequent rheumatic diseases. Rheumatic fever, traumatic and infectious arthritis (including Reiter's disease), and tumors of the joints are specifically excluded as properly being in the domain of other monographs. Except for gout, metabolic diseases with joint manifestations are also excluded. Finally, that set of syndromes called bursitis, tendinitis, fibrositis, and psychogenic rheumatism will not be dealt with because they are too vague and ill defined to have yet been subjected to epidemiologic study.

1.2 Epidemiology is the study of the distribution of disease and injury in populations. It uses quantitative methods for description and hypothesis testing. I believe that the epidemiology of rheumatic diseases has now come to the point beyond which there is no excuse for further simple prevalence surveys. There are now on record substantial descriptive studies of the major rheumatic diseases, but to date there has been far too little hypothesis-testing and sophisticated analysis of the data already collected. One of the attempts of this monograph will be to show that there are more hypotheses and conclusions to be drawn from the available data than had been previously supposed.

1.3 Painful Swelling of Joints is the common denominator of arthritis. As Ropes and Bauer (1953) ably pointed out, much can be learned about the disease responsible for the painful swelling by examination of the joint fluid. While joint paracentesis is not a procedure that seems likely to become acceptable for field studies, X-rays of joints are acceptable except where they involve unreasonable risk to the gonads. They have provided useful information, particularly since the development of the *Atlas of Standard Radiographs of Arthritis* (1963).

By and large in the study of arthritis, the diseases must be classified not just by the nature and distribution of the joint response, which is really rather limited in its variety, but also by the associated manifestations in other systems. For example, gout is now acknowledged to be a metabolic disease with incidental and intermittent joint manifestations. Furthermore, the term "rheumatoid disease" is attaining more widespread usage than "rheumatoid arthritis" and the disease is becoming recognized without, as well as with, arthritis. In fact, possible diagnostic criteria for nonarticular rheumatoid disease were proposed at the Rome conference in 1961 (Kellgren *et al.*, 1963).

1.4 The Principle of Severity Gradient. Infectious disease epidemiologists have come to assume the importance of recognizing the shape of the distribution of disease along its severity gradient. In Figure 1.1 are shown three such frequency distributions by severity. The cases of human rabies pile up at the fatal end of the distribution, while diphtheria is a disease that has many subclinical infections, and measles is a disease with few attenuated cases and few deaths but many cases of moderate severity. Epidemiologists are aware that immunization against diphtheria does not prevent infection but does produce a marked shift of the cases toward the mild end of the severity gradient.

The importance of the full range of the severity gradient was recognized in the development of the diagnostic criteria for rheumatoid arthritis (Ropes *et al.*, 1957) and in the development of criteria for radiologic diagnosis (*Atlas of Standard Radiographs,* 1963), but it has not received as much attention as it deserves in the reporting of surveys. The certainty of diagnosis is clearly related to the severity of the disease: while one may recognize a classic crippling case of rheumatoid disease as the patient walks in the door, it may take many visits to classify a mild case.

1.5 Remittency. A related problem is the fact that the severe cases are usually continuously active cases, while the mild ones are only intermittently active and cannot be classified until an exacerbation takes place. This means that there is a built-in underestimate of the frequency of the mildest cases. A theoretically sound but practically difficult method for dealing with this phenomenon has been proposed (Beall and Cobb, 1961; Cobb, 1962). This method uses sequential surveys of a population to obtain increments in newly discovered cases from one survey to the next. From these increments

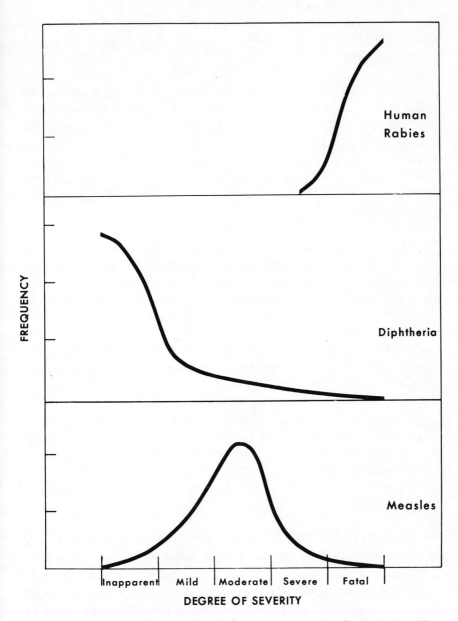

Fig. 1.1 Illustrative frequency distributions by degree of severity: rabies, diphtheria and measles compared.

the moments of the distribution and hence the distribution according to proportion of time in episode can be calculated. It seems likely that this method will be used more as the need to understand the full gradient of these diseases increases.

1.6 Pain is all too commonly the guide to decisions about the care with which a person's joints are examined and about which joints should receive the most attention. It has been a frequent observation in the training of field observers that initially they will overreport swelling in painful or tender joints and underreport it in pain-free joints. This is not surprising, but it raises some interesting questions about bias in the diagnosis of arthritis in favor of those most likely to complain.

We need to know much more about pain and its causes, for example, Why do some people with osteoarthrosis have pain while others with equally severe involvement do not?, or Of all the people with spondylolisthesis, what characterizes the small number who have pain?, or Is the greater frequency of mild rheumatoid arthritis in Jamaica more a complaint-bias phenomenon than a real phenomenon? We need to understand better who overreports and who underreports pain. Clearly, a lot of cultural factors are involved and they may influence patterns of reporting by age and sex (Lawrence and Aitken-Swan, 1952; Zborowski, 1952).

1.7 Age-Sex Adjustment. It is obvious that there are very large differences in the frequency of the rheumatic diseases by age and sex, yet one still finds in the literature comparisons between populations that are not specific with regard to age and sex, nor adjusted for age and sex, nor even checked to see that the populations are of reasonably similar age-sex composition.

1.8 Etiology. The diseases of concern in this monograph by and large are diseases of unknown etiology. It behooves us then to be both flexible in our view of classification and eclectic in our approach to etiology. Most people would agree that ultimately classification should be on the basis of etiology. Since this is not possible at the moment, we must be prepared to revise our classification as our understanding of etiology improves.

On the face of it, this is a logical and sound position. But what of multifactorial etiology? Take, for example, the case of childhood asthma, which is generally conceded to receive causal contributions from both allergy and emotional disturbance in varying proportions. Occasionally one sees attacks that appear to be caused entirely by allergy or entirely by emotional disturbance. Should one give these attacks different names? It seems likely that we will be facing this kind of situation with regard to rheumatoid disease and perhaps with regard to other rheumatic diseases. It is my hope that as that time arrives, this field that has had more than its share of fashions and nostrums will become accepting of the notion of multifactorial etiology and of the possible need for new diagnostic rubrics.

1.9 History. Concern over the magnitude of the problem of the rheumatic diseases is by no means new. Socrates placed arthritis first in a list of the three commonest diseases of his time, and Diocletian passed an edict exempting Romans with severe arthritis from the payment of taxes (Burbank, 1943). Actual data collection began in the 1920's with the collection of some medical-care statistics (Kahlmeter, 1923; Ministry of Health of Great Britain, 1924, and 1928). This and other knowledge up to the end of the third decade of this century was well summarized by Glover (1930) in his Milroy lectures.

In 1936, a large-scale survey by district nurses was conducted in Finland (Holsti and Rantasalo, 1936). A few years later, a field study by specially trained medical students was reported from Sweden (Edström, 1944). Probably the first two fully medical surveys of rheumatic disease were done by Finns, the first in Finland itself (Holsti and Huuskonen, 1938) and the second in Greenland (Ehrström, 1951). Then in the early fifties, a series of systematic population studies was initiated by Lawrence at the Rheumatism Research Center in Manchester, England, and by Cobb in Pittsburgh, Pennsylvania. The need for diagnostic criteria was soon seen (Cobb *et al.,* 1955) and promptly met with regard to rheumatoid arthritis by the work of a committee of the American Rheumatism Association (Ropes *et al.,* 1957). The first international comparison based on these criteria was published in the same year (Cobb and Lawrence, 1957).

Since 1957, there has developed an ever-growing list of population surveys for rheumatic disease in Europe, North America, New Zealand, Australia, the Middle East, and Japan. Now that the past decade has laid the foundations and developed the techniques, the next decade should produce some important epidemiology of the rheumatic diseases.

2 / RHEUMATIC COMPLAINTS

2.0 Introduction. The full extent of the rheumatism problem is not demonstrated by reports of diagnosable rheumatic disease. As every practitioner knows, a large proportion of persons seeking treatment for rheumatic disease have conditions that are not assignable with any confidence to one or another of the rheumatic-disease categories. Furthermore, Kellgren and his associates (1953) found that about 50 percent of persons with rheumatic complaints in Leigh, England, had never consulted a physician about these complaints. Lincoln and Cobb (1963) had approximately the same findings among maintenance workers in Oak Ridge, Tennessee, so it seems appropriate to conclude that rheumatic complaints are generally not viewed as very serious and are therefore subject to appreciable underreporting. Furthermore, the episodic nature of most of the milder rheumatic conditions permits memory defects to further reduce the proportion of rheumatism-sufferers who can be identified by one or another technique. With these thoughts in mind, let us examine the various possible ways of assessing the general magnitude of the rheumatism problem.

2.1 Sources of Data. There are many ways of estimating the impact of disease on a population. Certainly mortality is an important criterion, and for many conditions the mortality rate or the extent to which life expectancy would be extended if the disease in question were to be completely eliminated is the most relevant measure. In dealing with the rheumatic diseases this is not the case, for here we have a situation in which mortality is low and morbidity is high. Table 2.1 indicates that the ratio of persons dying in a year to persons reporting themselves as permanently disabled is only 1:20, to persons having an illness of seven days or longer is 1:200, and to persons complaining of rheumatism is about 1:2,000. Although these figures are not derived from strictly comparable populations and it is not possible to adjust for age and sex, they are close enough to show the scale on which the severity gradient is measured.

With a gradient as extensive as this, one naturally needs a variety of points to describe it fully. In order of decreasing severity the following points suggest themselves:

    (a) Total disability
    (b) Partial or intermittent disability
    (c) Medical treatment
    (d) Complaints, total and medically verifiable.

6

Table 2.1　Severity gradient of rheumatism
in the United States, 1936

Measure	Rate per 1,000 persons
Mortality rate (U.S. Bureau of Census, 1938)	0.03
Prevalence of permanent orthopedic impairments due to rheumatism (Britten et al., 1940)	0.8
Annual prevalence of illness of 7 days or longer due to rheumatism (Britten et al., 1940)	5.9
Prevalence of persons who complain of rheumatism on household survey (Hailmen, 1941)	47.5

2.2 Total Disability. Definitions vary from one study to another, but for the United States there are two bits of data, quite disparate in definition, that give roughly the same frequency estimates. The first is the figure of 0.8 per 1,000 with permanent orthopedic impairments caused by rheumatism, as noted in Table 2.1. The second is the figure of 1.1 per 1,000 with major mobility limitation (U.S. National Health Survey, 1960*b*). Neither figure includes those persons in institutions for the chronically ill. The fact that one person in 10,000 received some allowance for arthritis under the U.S. Old Age, Survivors, and Disability Insurance plan in 1962 does not help, for the eligibility requirements for certification are so restrictive that they exclude all but a small percentage of the disabled (U.S. Public Health Service, 1966).

Data from other countries suggest the same order of magnitude. Kalbak (1953) reports that roughly one person in 1,000 receives public aid in Denmark each year because ability to work has been reduced to less than one-third of normal by a rheumatic disease. In 1936 Holsti and Rantasalo estimated on the basis of a survey that 2.5 per 1,000 were "totally disabled" by chronic rheumatism in Finland. For Japan in 1952, Shichikawa and his co-workers (1966) report that 0.3 per 1,000 received government support because of rheumatoid or tuberculous arthritis.

With these facts in mind, a working estimate of one per thousand appears to be the right order of magnitude for the prevalence of total disability resulting from arthritis and rheumatism, although better estimates are overdue. In fact, it might be appropriate to establish local registers of the really disabled to make sure that they receive the care they need. From such registers the demographic and diagnostic characteristics of severely disabled arthritics might also be determined. Clearly, survey methods are too expensive for the study of conditions as rare as this.

2.3 Partial Disability. There are many counts of the number of people who have had disabling illness for specified periods of time. One of the more common durations is the industrial insurance cut-off of eight days or more. A convenient example of the data comes from the Metropolitan Life Insurance Company and is presented in Table 2.2. As can be seen, women are more affected than men, and the rates increase with age.

These figures really give only one point on a continuum of severity. Perhaps a better overall picture is obtained when we think of arthritis as accounting for something between 9 and 15 percent of days lost from work (Brown and Lingg, 1961; Anderson *et al.,* 1962; Anderson and Duthie, 1963). In Great Britain, rheumatism shares the top of the list of diseases causing time lost from work with chronic bronchitis (Tegner, 1964). In the United States, it is second only to heart disease (U.S. Public Health Service, 1966).

Table 2.2   Annual incidence per 1,000 of arthritis disabling for 8 days or more in personnel of the Metropolitan Life Insurance Company for two time periods

Age	1953-55		1965	
	M	F	M	F
25-34	0.6	2.0	0.8	1.8
35-44	2.2	4.2	0.8	2.4
45-54	2.6	5.9	2.5	5.8
55-59	5.6	14.1	6.5	8.3
60-64	8.8	-		

Source: Metropolitan Life Insurance Company, 1956 and 1967.

Table 2.3   Days of disability per 1,000 persons per year due to arthritis and rheumatism as reported in household interviews in the United States, July 1957 - June 1959

Age group	Restricted activity			Bed disability		
	Total	Males	Females	Total	Males	Females
25-44	485	292	662	148	129	166
45-64	2788	1987	3542	691	498	873
65 +	7858	6098	9334	1960	1484	2359

Source: U.S. National Health Survey, 1960b.

Table 2.3 shows the number of days of restricted activity and bed disability per 1,000 persons of specified age and sex as estimated from household interviews in the U.S. National Health Survey (1960b). The restricted-activity data are about in line with the actual industrial experience of working men in Scotland reported by Anderson and Duthie (1963) and Anderson et al. (1962), and are remarkably close to the number of days of sickness reported in the practitioner's inquiry, (Ministry of Health of Great Britain, 1924). This gives us confidence that the data presented in the table constitute appropriate and useful estimates.

2.4 Medical Treatment. From the data presented by Avnet in her very useful book (1967), the figures in Table 2.4 have been derived. Anyone with a slide rule can quickly verify that while rheumatic complaints account for 8 percent of the cases seen by physicians, these diagnoses account for only 4.1 percent of the office visits, 2.9 percent of the consultations, and 1.3 percent of the hospitalizations. On the other hand, they do account for 7.7 percent of the diagnostic X-rays taken outside the hospital. The division into arthritis and rheumatism; synovitis, bursitis, and tenosynovitis; and pain in the back is presented to show how the totals were derived. It should be clear that the counts are of services, not people receiving service.

The total services provided for arthritis and related conditions in this study in New York seem to compare fairly well with the data from the Province of Ontario, Canada, even though direct comparisons cannot be made because of differences in the composition of the groups and in the methods of counting services (le Riche et al., 1965b).

Table 2.4 Medical care for arthritis and related conditions compared to total medical care for Group Health Insurance

Services	Rates per 1,000 insured population per year				
	Total for all illnesses	Total for rheumatic complaints	Arthritis, rheumatism	Synovitis, bursitis, tenosynovitis	Pain in back
Cases	802.0	64.1	30.3	28.2	5.6
Office visits	3522.5	143.5	75.6	61.3	6.6
GP		108.6	57.5	46.2	4.9
Specialist		34.9	18.1	15.1	1.7
Home visits	804.4	12.6	6.6	5.6	0.4
Office surgery	157.3	6.4	1.2	4.9	0.3
Consultation	77.8	2.3	0.8	1.2	0.3
Diagnostic X-rays[a]	202.6	15.6	7.4	6.4	1.8
Laboratory tests[a]	693.4	15.9	11.4	3.6	0.9
Hospitalizations	114.0	1.5	0.4	1.0	0.1
Hospital days	851.0	10.5	5.8	4.3	0.4

Source: Avnet, 1967.

[a] Services provided while in hospital not included.

On the other hand, to the extent that comparisons can be made, it would appear that consultations or physician visits for arthritis and rheumatism are substantially more frequent under the British National Health Service (Logan and Cushion, 1958). Hospitalizations for arthritis and rheumatism would seem to be somewhat more frequent in Ontario (le Riche *et al.,* 1965*a*) and especially in Saskatchewan (Saskatchewan Department of Health, 1966).

Finally, one must never forget that arthritics characteristically shop around for advice and many of them get into the hands of nonmedical practitioners. No recent estimates of the frequency of this have been uncovered but the data of Collins (1940) suggests that about one-third of all the calls on practitioners for rheumatism and related diseases are on nonmedical practitioners, whereas only about 10 percent of the calls for all other causes are on nonmedical practitioners. This is a matter that deserves further serious attention in terms of up-to-date information and the reasons for the phenomenon. It is a significant area on which those of us interested in improving care for the arthritic have too often turned our backs.

From other sources we find that some form of arthritis or rheumatism is the primary diagnosis for 6.5 percent of adults in nursing homes in Maryland in 1952 and results in 4.6 percent of the morbidity visits made by the Baltimore (Maryland) Visiting Nurse Association in 1953 (Perrott *et al.*, 1954). It is also the reason for an approximately equal proportion of visiting-nurse services supplied by the Health Insurance Plan of Greater New York (1961), and is the principal diagnosis of 2.3 percent of the patients in a group of four chronic-disease hospitals (Goldman, 1962).

2.5 Complaints. Unfortunately, complaint data from various sources are not really very comparable. For example, Table 2.5 demonstrates the relationship between a household-survey report of arthritis or rheumatism, an individual report of arthritis or rheumatism, and the result of a medical examination of the same 429 individuals 15 years of age and older from Pittsburgh, Pennsylvania. The population has been converted to 1,000 for easy perception of rates.

Table 2.5 The distribution of persons by gradient of arthritis and classification on certain questions about arthritis and rheumatism , lifetime prevalence rates per 1,000 persons 15 years of age and over for the Arsenal Health District of Pittsburgh, 1952 to 1954

Physician classification	Household survey report of arthritis or rheumatism			Individual interview report of arthritis or rheumatism	
	Total	Yes	No [a]	Yes	No [a]
Total responses	1,000	75	925	209	791
Classical arthritis	71	21	50	42	29
Definite arthritis	147	24	123	82	65
Rheumatic complaints	101	19	82	44	57
Questionable complaints	262	9	253	40	222
No suspicion of arthritis	419	2	417	1	418

Source: Cobb et al., 1956.

[a] "Don't know" answers, amounting to about 1 percent of the total, have been included here.

It is amusing that the prevalence of classical arthritis is 71 per 1,000 and the prevalence of household-survey reports of arthritis is 75 per 1,000. Likewise the prevalence of classical plus definite arthritis is 71 + 147 = 218 per 1,000 while the prevalence of "yes" reports on the individual interview is 209 per 1,000. For clarification it is worth noting that in this instance classical arthritis refers to any case that fits the classical description of the relevant type of arthritis, whatever that might have been. On the other hand, definite arthritis refers to any case having had a well-defined episode of nontraumatic joint disease without regard to whether it could be placed in a specific diagnostic category.

From the body of the table it is apparent that this correspondence is largely a result of chance. Specifically, the persons found by the physician to have classical arthritis for whom a positive response was given in the household survey were only 21 per 1,000, or less than one-third of the total. With the individual interview the overlap is considerably larger, for 42 + 82 = 124 persons out of the 218 who had either classical or definite arthritis responded positively to the question. Despite the fact that the household interviews antedated the examinations by about a year and the individual interviews antedated the examinations by about a month, these results make us cautious about the interpretation of interview data.

It is important to note that 71 + 147 + 101 = 318 per 1,000, or 32 percent of this random sample of an urban population 15 years of age and older, complained to the examining physician. These complaints, however, did not necessarily lead to a diagnosis and were only verifiable in less than two-thirds of the cases. In addition, there were 262 per 1,000 who had complaints that the physician doubted were really rheumatic in origin.

At this point one might quite properly throw up one's hands and say that there is no such thing as a meaningful estimate of the frequency of rheumatic complaints. However, there are some surprising regularities in the data which are worthy of note. First, there are six surveys in North America that have given household-survey prevalence rates between 45 and 95 per 1,000 for arthritis and rheumatism (Hailman, 1941; Woolsey, 1952; Cobb *et al.*, 1956; Canada, Bureau of Statistics, 1960; U.S. National Health Survey, 1960*b*; U.S. Public Health Service, 1966). The lowest rate of 47.5 was obtained in the National Health Survey of 1936 which included few people over 65 years of age (Hailman, 1941). The usual inquiries covered all illnesses, with a reminder list of chronic conditions including arthritis and rheumatism, but the two highest rates (Woolsey, 1952; Cobb, 1956) were the result of the question "Does any member of this household have arthritis or rheumatism?" So we see that although the household survey produces considerable underreporting, there is a substantial agreement from one survey to the next.

The one recent household survey that appears out of line is the one done in Hawaii for which the rate is only 22 per 1,000 (U.S. National Health Survey, 1960a). The situation in Hawaii deserves further investigation to explain this difference.

The second indication of uniformity in the frequency of rheumatic complaints is presented in Table 2.6. Here are given figures from a series of surveys in this country and others, each adjusted to age 14 or 15 and over and to exclude rheumatic fever. The Pittsburgh data include a history of joint swelling and/or a finding of pain on motion or tenderness in some joint. The rate has been adjusted for nonresponse bias. The National Health Survey data are taken from the

Table 2.6 The frequency of medically verified rheumatic complaints in three surveys in the United States compared with studies in other countries

Survey Location	Rate per 1,000 [a]
Civilian non-institutionalized population, age 15 + Baltimore, Md. (Commission on Chronic Illness, 1957)	210
Civilian non-institutionalized population, age 15 + Pittsburgh, Pa. (Cobb, 1956)	190
Civilian non-institutionalized population, age 18-79 USA (National Center for Health Statistics, 1966c)	170
England (Kellgren et al, 1953)	190
Netherlands (de Blécourt and Basart, 1953)	180
Czechoslovakia (Sitaj et al, 1954)	130
Australia (Nelson and Lancaster, 1959)	230
Japan (Shichikawa et al, 1966)	160

[a] The rates have been adjusted where necessary by removal of rheumatic fever and deletion of persons under 14 or 15 and have been rounded to two significant figures. A proper age adjustment is not possible on these data.

appendix of the report on rheumatoid arthritis and include any person who had at least one positive finding on physical examination.

The difference in the rates may be accounted for by the inclusion of historical information about swelling in the Pittsburgh study. The other studies are done in reasonably comparable fashion, but for the most part are not as well defined in the relevant publications. The somewhat lower prevalence in Czechoslovakia results from the fact that the sample was appreciably younger than elsewhere.

The tabulation looks impressive, and its consistent nature gives a feeling that something solid has been measured. However, one is forced to marvel at this consistency in view of the extraordinary variation from plant to plant within one company found by Densen and his co-workers (1955). If all future surveys were to follow the lead of the National Center for Health Statistics (1966c) and publish relevant details in an appendix, comparability would be materially improved. The reader is cautioned to remember that the inclusion of all complaints mentioned by a subject to the examining physician may nearly double the rates. Also, the desirability of proper age-sex adjustments should be emphasized. Unfortunately, several of the above reports did not present breakdowns which would make such adjustments possible.

2.6 Effects of Age, Sex, and Heavy Work. Figure 2.1 shows that whatever measure is used, the rates of rheumatic affliction increase with age. In this arith-log plot, comparisons of slope can be made visually. It is interesting to note that the upper curves involving human response to the conditions gradually fall off at ages past 55, while the destruction of joints with limitation of mobility proceeds inexorably with advancing years.

Table 2.7 shows the sex ratios for various degrees of severity of arthritis and rheumatism. It is striking that the male-to-female ratio is about 0.5 for all the mild and moderate degrees of involvement, but when it comes to major limitation of activity the ratio suddenly jumps to 1.2. The meaning of this phenomenon is not immediately clear and deserves further study. It may result partially from the usual reluctance of men in Western culture to complain or give in to modest afflictions. In further support of this point it should be noted that the number of days lost to arthritis and rheumatism per working person per year is exactly the same for the two sexes. This indicates that the excess of women over men with bed disability must be accounted for by women who are not employed.

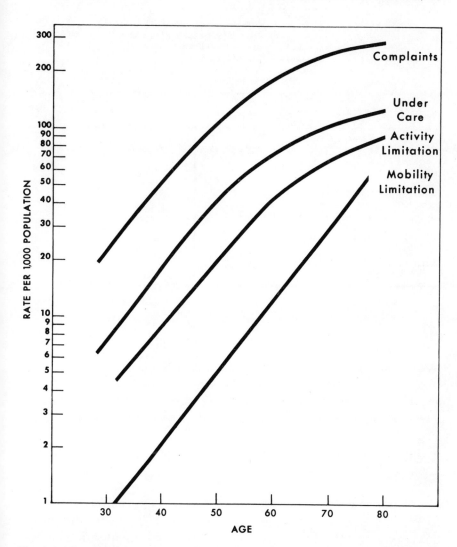

Fig. 2.1 The prevalence per 1,000 persons by age of various degrees of severity of rheumatic affliction as reported in household interviews, United States, July 1957 to June 1959, based on 73,000 interviews. (U.S. National Health Survey, 1960*b*.)

From many sources, particularly Sappington (1924), Danichewsky (1932), Lawrence and Aitken-Swan (1952), Anderson and Duthie (1963), the U.S. Public Health Service (1966), and Lawrence *et al.* (1966*d*), there is evidence that those who engage in heavy physical work outdoors, especially farming, have more total arthritis than those who do light work indoors. Observed urban-rural differences,

Table 2.7   Number of persons per 1,000 with various
degrees of severity of arthritis and
rheumatism as reported in household
interviews by sex, with sex ratios

Severity	M	F	Ratio M/F
With complaints	46.1	80.7	.57
Under care	15.9	33.9	.47
With 1+ days bed disability per year	5.0	9.3	.54
With 7+ days bed disability per year	3.2	5.7	.56
With mobility limitation	4.2	8.8	.48
With major activity limitation per 1,000	3.7	3.0	1.22

Source: U.S. National Health Survey, 1960b.

Negro-white differences, and social-class differences have to be controlled for type of work before the surveys can be assumed to have any meaning beyond this. It should be remembered that those in the lower social classes do more heavy work, have more arthritis, and are less liable to get adequate medical care. Therefore, the largest group of those needing treatment for arthritis is in the lowest socioeconomic class.

   2.7 Overview. Arthritis and rheumatism are important as sources of complaints and causes of lost time from work. These conditions do not appear to get a proportionate share of medical attention and do seem to get an undue share of the attention of nonmedical practitioners. Rheumatic complaints increase in frequency with age and heavy outdoor work.

3 / THE FREQUENCY OF
RHEUMATOID DISEASE

3.0 Introduction. In treating the subject of rheumatoid disease, it is important to remember that we are dealing with a systemic disease that involves the mesenchymal connective tissue at a wide variety of sites (Bauer and Clark, 1948; Dresner, 1955; Sever, 1965). To date it has seldom been diagnosed without arthritis. Perhaps the most urgent research need is to develop ways of recognizing rheumatoid disease without arthritis, which I suspect is much more common than most of us would believe. Until this problem is unraveled, we shall have to continue to study the epidemiology of rheumatoid arthritis, which is surely only a portion – and possibly a quite atypical portion – of the disease.

A second bias in the study of rheumatoid disease stems from its mild and intermittent nature. The mild cases are seldom seen by a physician; those of intermediate severity are seen by the general practitioner and the general internist; only the most severe cases are seen by the consulting rheumatologist. I would estimate that the consulting rheumatologist sees about one-fifteenth of the existing probable rheumatoids, one-fifth of the definite cases, and nearly all of the classical cases. This gives the consultant a biased view of the relative frequency of cases by degree of severity, thereby limiting progress in the field and tending to restrict the diagnosis to more severe, progressive, and disabling forms of the disease.

It is my belief that if this disease is to be understood, we must direct our attention to the full extent of the severity gradient. It is important to remember that poliomyelitis was not understood until after it was recognized that there were perhaps 100 nonparalytic infections for every crippling case. If we exclude such a possibility from our thinking by narrow definitions of rheumatoid disease, we may put off the time when its evolution and distribution in the population will be fully comprehended.

A third issue of importance is the fact that rheumatoid disease may turn out to be a group of diseases. At least in field studies, which are so expensive, it is therefore important to collect the data in such a way that they can be reanalyzed at a later date if new discoveries suggest better methods of classification.

With these disclaimers let us turn to what is known about the classification and frequency of rheumatoid arthritis.

3.1 Diagnostic Criteria. Criteria for the diagnosis of a disease need to set boundaries laterally between diseases and horizontally across the severity gradient to establish the point below which the cases will be considered too mild to be counted. It is useful to remember several points when working with diagnostic criteria:

(a) The severity of a disease and the security with which one can make the diagnosis are strongly related.

(b) For any disease, classification will remain inadequate until the etiology is known. It is extremely important to continue striving for etiologic classification rather than adhering to old rubrics that merely have prognostic or therapeutic significance.

(c) With any classification dimension, as one shifts the cutting point there are reciprocal changes in sensitivity and specificity. This is by no means a new insight and has been well discussed by Horvath (1964). It means that there are two ways to assemble a set of criteria. The first is to put sensitive criteria together with "and's." The second is to put specific criteria together with "or's." Of the two, the first is preferable because the set of criteria linked with "and's" has the useful property of being quite sensitive when only one or two criteria are met and highly specific when many have been met.

(d) It is generally recognized that for a set of criteria one wants manifestations that are reliably observable. However, if one has a set of manifestations on each of which there is a probability of overclassification of, say 0.15, the probability of gross overclassification of the individual decreases as the number of criteria fulfilled increases. For example, if an individual is reported to meet five criteria, the probability that he has been simultaneously misclassified on three of the dimensions — that is, that in reality he does not truly meet a total of three criteria — is $(0.15)^3$ or 0.003. By the same token, the use of multiple observers can substantially reduce classification error.

The relevance of these basic points about classification will become apparent to the reader as he progresses through this and subsequent sections.

Classification with respect to rheumatoid arthritis began with the Stage of Disease and the Class of Functional Impairment suggested by Steinbrocker and his committee in 1949. In 1956, Ropes and her committee of the American Rheumatism Association (Ropes *et al.,* 1957) proposed a set of criteria that took into account separation from other diseases as well as cut-off points on the severity gradient. In 1958, these proposed criteria were revised (Ropes *et al.*, 1959) into a form that has been the basis for most of the epidemiologic work in the subsequent ten years.

These criteria have been commented on by a variety of investigators; as expected, there is general agreement that they fall short of perfection. The relevant literature has been summarized by Cobb (1960) and Abramson (1967). The most serious criticisms of the criteria fall into two more or less opposing categories. There is one point of view that says the criteria are too restrictive, and that what really is needed is the addition of two sets of criteria, one for inactive disease and one for nonarticular disease. This point of view predominated in the Second International Symposium on Population Studies in Relation to Chronic Rheumatic Diseases held in Rome in 1961 (Kellgren, 1962; Kellgren *et al.*, 1963).

Quite a different point of view was in ascendancy, though not agreed to by all, at the Third International Symposium held in New York in 1966 (Bennett and Burch, 1967). This view emphasizes the likelihood that the 1958 criteria include more than one disease, and that nodule-forming seropositive disease is quite different from the rest of the syndrome. Those holding this point of view believe that the term *rheumatoid arthritis* should be limited to "a syndrome that a clinical rheumatologist would diagnose as R.A. in a patient seeking professional advice" (Kellgren, 1968). This is a clinical point of view that neglects the less visible part of the severity gradient and therefore is not really sound epidemiology as has been pointed out by the distinguished epidemiologic thinker, John Gordon (1950).

However one views the details, the fact remains that criteria have been developed and attempts are being made to improve them. Their use has made it possible to compare population studies done in different places and at different times. The criteria recommended at the Third International Symposium on Population Studies of the Rheumatic Diseases are as follows (Bennett and Burch, 1967):

1. A history, past or present, of an episode of joint pain involving three or more limb joints, without stipulation as to duration. For the purposes of this criterion, the joints on either side shall count separately, but joints that occur in groups (e.g. the PIPs or MCPs on one side) shall count only as a single joint, even if more than one of them is involved on the same side.
2. Involvement by swelling, limitation, subluxation or ankylosis of at least three limb joints (excluding the DIPs, the fifth PIPs, the first carpometacarpal [CMC] joints, the hips and the first MTPs) with symmetry of at least one joint pair. There must be involvement of one hand, wrist or foot,

as involvement limited to large joints such as elbows or knees does not satisfy this criterion. Subluxation of the lateral MTPs must be irreducible.
3. X-ray features of grade 2 or more erosive arthritis in the hands, wrists or feet.
4. Positive serological reaction for rheumatoid (anti-gamma globulin) factor, determined by a method that is controlled by periodic testing of reference sera and by exchange of sera with other laboratories.

Joint Score. A joint score should be applied to those meeting, for example, two or more of the criteria for RA. A score of one is given for each limb joint involved clinically, with exclusions as in criterion #2 and counting each joint group, e.g. PIPs, as one joint, scoring each side separately.

Components for the joint score (one for each side). 2nd-4th PIPs, MCPs, intracarpals, wrists, elbows and shoulders. IPs of toes, 2nd-5th MTPs, tarsals, subtaloids, ankles, knees and neck (one point). Possible maximum = 25.

Recommendations for summation of the criteria for polyarthritis and RA were not made and were considered unnecessary so long as the distribution of each criterion was reported individually. However, concordance of the criteria should be reported, particularly that between clinical criteria for polyarthritis and RA and radiological and serological findings.

3.2 Validity and Reproducibility of the Clinical Criteria. The only really thoughtful study of the validity of the clinical criteria known to me is the admirable paper of Abramson (1967). It should be studied with care by everyone concerned with this problem. Abramson not only reviews the data from several sources, but analyzes them in various ways. His conclusion that the clinical criteria are more valid than the X-ray and laboratory criteria is amply justified. The demonstration that his material from Jerusalem gives a clean Guttman scale for the six clinical criteria is eloquent support for the work of the ARA Committee on Diagnostic Criteria (Ropes *et al.,* 1957).

On the subject of reproducibility, little information is available. Data of this sort are difficult to come by because on the whole people who volunteer for a survey do not care to be examined successively by two different physicians at the same visit. Furthermore, the disease is remittent, which means that intervals of more than a few days may lead to changes interpretable as disagreement between observers.

Some years ago at Oak Ridge, Tennessee, I investigated the effect of the interval between examinations and found that agreement did not decrease appreciably until the interval exceeded eight days. O'Sullivan and his colleagues in Sudbury, Massachusetts (1968) did two examinations on the same day. The results from the two studies are presented in Table 3.1

Table 3.1   Agreement between observers as percent of total reported
             positive by either observer at independent examinations

	Two physicians same day Sudbury, Mass.[a]	Physician and nurse within eight days Oak Ridge, Tenn.[b]
Joint swelling	27%	61%
Tenderness or pain on motion	47%	73%
Morning stiffness	-	67%
No. of paired examinations	547	350

[a] O'Sullivan, Cathcart and Bolzan, 1968.
[b] Cobb, unpublished.

In the Oak Ridge study, a great deal of effort went into reducing
interobserver variation, and it is clear that results better than those
obtained by O'Sullivan and his colleagues can be managed. It is my
belief that this source of error can be reduced even further by frequent examinations with two examiners present, followed by discussion of the findings. As evidence for this, two trends were found
in analysis of the Oak Ridge interobserver variation data. First, the
agreement between myself and the nurse whom I trained was appreciably better than the agreement between the nurse and the three
industrial physicians who received only general guidance in the con-
duct of a joint examination. Second, the agreement appeared to
improve with time.

A further way to reduce the errors introduced by observer variation
is to insist on double evaluation of every person with three or more
criteria positive, and of a sample of those persons who do not have
three positive findings. Such double examinations should ideally be
followed by a conference with the patient present so that differences
of opinion can be reconciled. This technique was used in the Oak
Ridge studies (Beall and Cobb, 1961; Lincoln and Cobb, 1963), and
no case was designated as rheumatoid arthritis unless the nurse and at
least one, and usually two, physicians agreed that joint swelling was
present. When two physicians had examined the individual and dis-
agreed as to the findings, further observations were made in subsequent months before the individual was accepted as having the
disease.

3.3 Validity and Reproducibility of the X-ray Criterion. The basic work on the validity of the X-ray criterion has been done by Kellgren and his group (Kellgren, 1956; Kellgren and Lawrence, 1957*b*; *Atlas of Standard Radiographs of Arthritis,* 1963). The most difficult problem has always been the evaluation of osteoporosis. The use of a control bone as advocated by Steven (1947) was the first step forward. Actual measurement of cortical thickness was introduced by Saville (1967) and should help considerably. Narrowing of joint space is not easily assessed unless it is very marked; in fact, some years ago I undertook to measure joint space and found that observer variation in measuring the same films, let alone different films of the same joint, was too great to warrant further effort. Likewise, it is almost impossible to make the distinction between a small bone cyst and a rheumatoid erosion for which the break in the cortex does not show. All this results in considerable observer variation in the reading of X-rays. For example, the agreement between observers in the Jerusalem survey (Abramson, 1967) on positives was only 3 out of 22, or 14 percent, which is considerably worse than the agreement on clinical findings. A similar level of agreement between Lawrence and myself occurred in reading a sample of X-rays from the Oak Ridge studies. Lawrence was involved in both studies; in both instances, his readings were less sensitive and more specific than those of the other readers. A somewhat higher degree of agreement is to be found within Kellgren's group (Kellgren, 1956), although the results are still not as reproducible as the clinical observations noted in Table 3.1.

Efforts are still being made to improve X-ray assessment in this disease (Berens *et al.,* 1968; Cathcart *et al.,* 1968) so we should not be discouraged. Those familiar with the problems of observer variation in radiology (Neyman, 1947; Etter *et al.,* 1960; and Lillienfeld and Kordan, 1966) are not surprised, but rather pleased that we are able to do so well. The results suggest strongly that double reading of X-rays in surveys for rheumatoid arthritis is important.

The value of X-ray examination as a diagnostic test for clinical rheumatoid arthritis is estimated in Table 3.2 from four studies in three countries. In no case does Youden's J exceed 25 percent for X-ray evaluation. However, with multiple readings, the staff of the U.S. Health Examination Survey were able to achieve a specificity of 99.7 percent (rounded in the table to 100 percent).

It is well to realize that the data presented in Table 3.2 are only moderately comparable. The difficulty, of course, is that in some of

Table 3.2   The diagnostic value for rheumatoid arthritis of X-ray,
serology and interview techniques. Selected data from
population samples

Test[a] and Author		Sensitivity[b]	Specificity[b]	J[b]
X-ray				
(Kellgren and Lawrence, 1956)		23%	93%	16%
(Ropes et al., 1957)		31	93	24
(DeGraaff, 1962)		17	83	0
(Abramson, 1967)		58	–	–
(Nat. Cent. Hlth. Stat., 1966c)		11	100	11
Serology				
DAT	(Kellgren and Lawrence, 1956)	23	97	20
SCAT	(Ball et al., 1962a)	15	98	13
SCAT	(Ball et al., 1962b)	0	98	-2
SCAT	(Valkenburg et al., 1966)	12	98	10
SCAT	(Bennett and Burch, 1968a)	29	94	23
LFT	(Mikkelsen et al., 1963)	26	98	24
LFT	(Valkenburg et al., 1966)	18	90	8
LFT	(Abramson, 1967)	44	96	40
BFT	(Nat. Cent. Hlth. Stat., 1966c)	20	97	13
BFT	(Bennett and Burch, 1968a)	37	90	27
PLAT	(Brooks and Cobb, 1963)	–	96	–
Interview				
RA Index	(Rubin et al., 1956)	66	95	61
RA Index	(Burch, 1964)	60	96	56
RA Index	(Burch, 1964)	58	95	53
RA Index	(Adler and Abramson, 1968)	41	93	34
RA Measure	(Cobb et al., 1969a)	86	98	84

Note: The definition of rheumatoid arthritis varies a little from
one study to another but not enough to invalidate the comparisons.

[a]DAT = Differential Agglutination Test; SCAT = Sheep Cell Agglutination Test; LFT = Latex Fixation Test; BFT = Bentonite Flocculation
Test; PLAT = Plate Latex Agglutination Test.

[b]

RA	Test		
	+	o	
+	a	b	a + b
o	c	d	c + d

Sensitivity = (a/a+b) 100

Specificity = (d/c+d) 100

$$J = \text{Sensitivity} + \text{Specificity} - 100$$
(Youden, 1950)

the early studies the diagnostic criteria were appreciably different
from the ARA criteria used in most of the studies — for example,
in the work of Kellgren and Lawrence (1956), Rubin *et al.* (1956),
Ropes *et al.* (1957), de Graaff (1962), and Mikkelsen *et al.* (1963).
With this limitation, plus the fact that the sample sizes are not always

large, one should be cautious about drawing detailed conclusions from these data. However, the general range of validity for the three techniques is well illustrated. It should be noted that sensitivity, specificity, and therefore also Youden's J are independent of the frequency of rheumatoid arthritis in the population under study.

3.4 Validity and Reproducibility of Serologic Tests. The serologic tests present a still more serious problem. Even though the reproducibility of most of the tests is excellent within a single laboratory, the variation between laboratories is appreciable (de Graaff, 1962; Nasou *et al.,* 1963; Schubart *et al.,* 1964). Persons with severe rheumatoid arthritis and high titers tend to remain positive indefinitely; still, the temporal stability of the titer is often only fair. This means that persons with low titer may shift back and forth with considerable frequency across the arbitrary boundary dividing positive from negative. This is true both in our own experience and in the experience of others (de Forest *et al.,* 1958; Ball and Lawrence, 1963; Schubart *et al.,* 1964).

The relationship between tests is indicated in Table 3.3. This table is not complete, but includes enough of the available data on population samples to indicate that the relationship between tests is at best rather weak. Agreement ranges from 12 to 57 percent of those positive on either test who are positive on both tests. In this connection it should be noted that interlaboratory agreement on the same test is sometimes no better than intralaboratory agreement between tests. In any case, there is difference enough between tests and between laboratories so that something is to be gained by doing multiple tests and checking the disagreements.

When one recognizes this lack of agreement between tests, it is not surprising that the relationship between a positive test and the diagnosis of rheumatoid arthritis has been very disappointing in population samples (Aho *et al.,* 1961; Ball *et al.,* 1962a and b; Ball and Lawrence, 1963; Mikkelsen *et al.,* 1963; Brooks and Cobb, 1964; Valkenburg *et al.,* 1966; Adler *et al.,* 1967b). Of course, in clinical samples these tests seem more useful because of the accumulation of persons with severe chronic rheumatoid arthritis. It has been said that these tests confirm obvious disease, but are of less help when the diagnosis is in doubt.

It seems clear that if the multiplicity of available tests are to become of any use to the epidemiologist, we must put a great deal of effort into seeking improved methods. The orderly exploration by Brooks and Cobb (1963) is one approach to the problem. However,

Table 3.3   The relationship between the more common tests[a] for rheumatoid factor in population samples; percent of those positive on either test who are positive on both tests

Test	PLAT	BFT	LFT	HEAT	RA-Test
SCAT	38	29	23		
		31[b]	45[c]	50[c]	
		40[d]	25[e]	56[e]	
		29[f]			
PLAT		41	45	14	20
BFT			57		
			52[e]		
LFT				38[c]	
				12[g]	
HEAT					17

Note: Those unmarked are population groups, size 130-140, done in my laboratory or in collaboration with my laboratory.

[a] HEAT = Human Erythrocyte Agglutination Test; RA-Test = Hyland Laboratories Slide Test; other abbreviations are as in Table 3.2

[b] Ball et al., 1962b.
[c] Ball et al., 1962a.
[d] Valkenburg, 1965.
[e] Valkenburg, et al., 1966.
[f] Bennett and Burch, 1968a.
[g] Adler et al., 1967b.

the stimulation provided by a series of interlaboratory comparisons, such as was done in testing for syphilis a generation ago, might be very worthwhile. If serology in this disease is not important enough to merit such comparisons, serologic testing in field studies may as well be abandoned for it contributes little to classification when competent radiology is available. I believe that with substantial effort better tests can be developed. I further believe that the process of developing these tests would contribute to better understanding of the disease in the same way that careful study of X-rays has contributed.

3.5 Interview Approaches. It should be perfectly clear that interview methods, and for that matter any imprecise measurement techniques, are useful primarily for detecting associations between the disease and various factors of interest (Rubin *et al.,* 1956; Mote and Anderson, 1965). Imprecise measures of any disease are useful in estimating its frequency if, and only if, one has exact knowledge of the proportion of false positives and the proportion of false negatives to be expected. Unfortunately, one can only have this knowledge with sufficient precision when the most valid method has been applied to the entire sample in question. In practice then, in order to estimate frequency it is necessary to do a study using clinical examinations, but in order to test hypotheses about associations that might have etiologic meaning, competent interview techniques may suffice. Incidentally, while we all acquire information by conversing with our associates, there is a great deal more to good interviewing than the average epidemiologist realizes (Kahn and Cannell, 1965; Survey Research Center, 1966).

Two interview measures have been utilized with some success. The first is the R.A. Index (Rubin *et al.,* 1956) which has now been used in a series of different populations. The several available estimates of sensitivity and specificity are presented in the last section of Table 3.2. The reduced specificity of the R.A. Index in Israel may result from its association with the tendency to complain that was found by Adler and Abramson (1968), along with the greater tendency to complain that is a cultural characteristic of their particular sample. For example, Adler and his associates (1967a) found the ratio of joint pain and tenderness to objective joint swelling to be four times as high as that for the United States. This is in line with differences between the cultures in response to pain (Zborowski, 1952) and therefore may be the proper interpretation of the data. In any case, the important conclusions are that validation of this type of index is not always transferable from one culture to another, and that in using indexes of this sort one must beware of the effects of the tendency to complain.

The second interview approach is much more ambitious and involves about forty questions repeated three times at intervals of several months (Cobb *et al.,* 1969a). This measure appears to have a sensitivity of 86 percent and a specificity of 98 percent, and is reasonably independent of the tendency to complain. It is so well within the range of between-physician variation in diagnosis that one is reminded of the old medical dictum that the history is the most important part of a medical workup. If this measure is to be used in other studies, further validation should be undertaken.

3.6 Relationships. The relationships among the major manifestations of rheumatoid disease have been a matter of continuing interest since the original call for diagnostic criteria (Cobb *et al.,* 1955). There are three areas in which findings occur: clinical, X-ray, and serologic. In each, there has been a tendency to want to sharpen the criteria by making them more restrictive. It is my opinion that we should focus instead on the reduction of observer variation. As we have seen, the best way to do this seems to involve more than one observer. It is easy to do more than one serologic test and to have the X-rays read by more than one radiologist, but it is not so easy, though equally important, to have multiple observations on borderline clinical findings.

Table 3.4 presents a comparable array of findings from the U.S. National Health Survey and from the British studies in Leigh and

Table 3.4   The relationship among the findings in two major surveys

Criteria	United States[a]			Great Britain[b]		
	Observed		Expected rate per 1,000	Observed		Expected rate per 1,000
	Number	Rate per 1,000		Number	Rate per 1,000	
Number examined	6,672			2,187		
At least one criterion	388	58		181	82	
3+ ARA clinical criteria	178	27		90	41	
Positive X-ray	42	6		46	21	
Positive serologic test[c]	206	31		90	41	
One and only one of the above	362	54		150	69	
Clinical and X-ray findings	16	2	0.2	22	10	0.9
Clinical and serologic findings	21	3	0.8	21	9	1.7
X-ray and serologic findings	15	2	0.2	16	7	0.9
Any two but not three	16	2	1.1	17	8	3.4
All three findings	12	2	0.005	14	6	0.04

[a] National Center for Health Statistics, 1966c.

[b] Kellgren, 1968.

[c] In U.S. Studies, BFT was used whereas in British studies SCAT was used.

Wensleydale. The only point on which the two are not quite comparable is the serologic test, for the Bentonite Flocculation Test was used in the United States and the Sheep-Cell Agglutination Test in Great Britain. Since the British data are taken from Kellgren's (1968) Table IV, they involve multiple X-ray readings like the American data. Our concern is with the fact seen in the last line that somewhere between 2 and 6 per 1,000 persons have clinical, radiological, and serologic evidence of rheumatoid arthritis. This is a rather small fraction of those meeting at least one criterion, in other words, 12 out of 388 and 14 out of 181. On the other hand, in each instance the frequency of those having all three positive bits of evidence is more than 100 times the expected number based on a random distribution of the findings in the population.

However you look at this group, it is important; for it contains the cases of severe progressive disease that commonly require rheumatologic consultation and hospitalization. They are the most visible and obvious cases, like the one-seventh of the iceberg that shows above the water. No one will quarrel with the diagnosis of rheumatoid arthritis in these cases, but many of us will quarrel with those who wish to limit the diagnosis to this highly visible segment of the severity gradient. As further research extends our knowledge, we will gradually be able to sharpen the boundaries of this disease in its less severe categories. For the time being, it is recommended that the published results of every survey include the detailed breakdown by patterns of manifestations provided as Appendix VI to the report by the National Center for Health Statistics (1966c).

3.7 Point Prevalence has been almost the only measure of frequency systematically applied to rheumatoid disease. As will be noted below, there are problems in making meaningful comparisons between populations using only the point prevalence. Furthermore, the age and sex differences are large enough so that comparisons require age-sex adjustment. To my knowledge, competent and appropriate adjustments have been made in only one report (Adler *et al.,* 1967a).

The data in Table 3.5 have been extracted from the more detailed Table 4.2 given later, in order to give the reader an immediate impression of the general frequency of rheumatoid arthritis in the middle years of life, from to 35 to 64. The range of 2 to 6 percent covers at least 90 percent of the point-prevalence studies that have been reported. There are some variations between groups that seem to be significant. These will be discussed in the next chapter.

Table 3.5   Age-sex adjusted[a] rates per 100 persons age 35–64
             for probable plus definite rheumatoid arthritis
             by A.R.A. criteria, from selected large studies

Study	Total	M	F
Israel	1.7	0.8	2.6
USA National Health Survey	3.0	1.7	4.4
Great Britain (Leigh & Wensleydale)	4.2	2.8	5.6
American Indians (Blackfeet & Pima)	5.1	4.5	5.8

Note: For sources and more detailed information about these and other studies, see Table 4.2.

[a] Adjusted to the U.S. population of 1940.

3.8 Incidence. Rheumatoid disease as a general rule does not have an abrupt onset. Even in those cases with a seemingly dramatic beginning, the careful history-taker usually finds that there have been mild episodes in the more remote past that seem insignificant beside the present illness. It is convenient and sensible to say that once a diagnosis of rheumatoid arthritis has been established there are no recoveries, only remissions of varying length. This suggests that incidence, which is the number of onsets per unit of population per unit of time, should be the appropriate measure of the disease frequency. Our inability to define and date an onset not only precludes doing the usual incidence studies, but also precludes calculating incidence from its relation to prevalence and duration, for estimation of duration is based on the time from onset to death.

However, there remain three possible approaches. The first involves the assumption that the prevalence and the population structure are reasonably constant through time. If this is so, the rheumatoid arthritics who are removed by death must exactly equal the number who are added by onsets. The mortality rate of persons with rheumatoid arthritis probably does not exceed 25 per 1,000 (Cobb *et al.*, 1953). If we assume a rough prevalence of 5 percent, or 500 per 10,000, we would expect $(25/1000) \times 500 = 12.5$ persons with rheumatoid arthritis per 10,000 population to die and 12.5 to take their place. In round numbers, let us say one new case per 1,000 population per year.

Now let us look at a quite different approach. In the study conducted at the Oak Ridge National Laboratory, keeping a group of employees under continuous observation for twenty-eight months (Lincoln and Cobb, 1963), the frequency of persons who at some time during the period had an episode meeting the ARA criteria for definite rheumatoid arthritis was just 5 percent. Most of these cases were mild and in a point-prevalence survey most would have been designated as possible or probable disease; a few would have been classified as entirely free of the disease.

In this study we were able to calculate the probability of moving from no disease to possible disease, from possible disease to probable disease, and from probable disease to definite disease. In each instance the probabilities turned out to be close to 0.18 per year. This incidence of 6 persons per 1,000 per year ($0.18 \times 0.18 \times 0.18 = 0.006$) would seem to be of the same order of magnitude as the previous estimate when one realizes that it refers to men in their working years rather than to the whole population, and that the estimate is probably additionally high because the study did not go on long enough to eliminate the discovery of pre-existing cases and confine itself to new onsets.

Another approach has been taken by Masi and his associates (1968). They have estimated the incidence of new diagnoses by physicians, which of course is not the same as the incidence of disease. (As will be noted in section 3.10, nearly half of the persons found to have rheumatoid arthritis on survey have not sought treatment for their disease.) Over a period of fifteen months Masi and his collaborators estimated the annual incidence of new diagnoses to be 2.8 per 1,000 for the nearly 1,000,000 people of Memphis and Shelby County, Tennessee.

Even though these several estimates have given us a rough approximation of the incidence of rheumatoid disease, it is felt that none of the methods is sufficiently reliable to use for epidemiologic purposes. In particular, Masi's method will be subject to all the biases inherent in his confounding of illness and illness behavior (Kasl and Cobb, 1964 and 1966).

3.9 Patterns of Manifestations over Time. A study of 331 men observed each month for sixteen months and then every four months for an additional year yielded clear evidence of the remittent nature of rheumatoid arthritis. Figure 3.1 shows a set of these patterns selected from a longitudinal study of employed men. Details of the

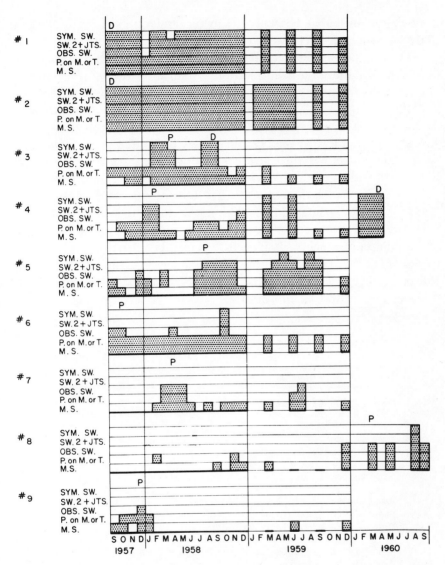

Fig. 3.1 Nine cases selected from the Oak Ridge (Tennessee) Arthritis Study to illustrate different symptom patterns over time. At the left margin are the ARA Criteria: M S = morning stiffness; P on M or T = pain on motion or tenderness; OBS SW = observed swelling: SW 2+JTS = swelling observed in two or more joints; SYM SW = symmetrical swelling. The superscripts P and D refer to the times at which diagnoses of probable or definite rheumatoid arthritis were made. Shading indicates that particular manifestation was present at that monthly screening. The heavy line at the bottom of each case is interrupted if that man was not screened in that month. (Reproduced with premission from Lincoln and Cobb, 1963.)

cases are presented elsewhere (Lincoln and Cobb, 1963). The first
five of the ARA criteria are shown on the vertical axis and the
relevant squares are shaded when the specified manifestations were
present for the month in question. *P* indicates the point at which a
diagnosis of probable disease was made and *D* denotes the time of a
definite diagnosis. The important thing to note about this figure is
that there is a wide variety of patterns: those at the top are continuously active, those at the bottom are symptom-free most of the time.

Table 3.6 shows the pattern of "progression" as these same men
were studied through time with one examination per month. It would
seem that this is a disease with slow transitions, for the table shows
that 120 men made 151 transitions. Of these 151 transitions, each
occurring in a month's time, only four are movements larger than to
the adjacent category. It is well to remember that the policy incor-
porated in the table is to maintain the highest classification achieved
even though a man with definite disease may have a remission that
leaves him entirely symptom free.

Table 3.6   The apparent progression of rheumatoid arthritis as observed in a group of 331 employed men
over a 28-month period

Progression of rheumatoid arthritis	Number of men
None to none	168
None to possible	77
None to possible to probable	14
None to possible to probable to definite	5
Possible to possible	30
Possible to probable	11
Possible to probable to definite	7
Probable to probable	1
Probable to definite	2
Definite to definite	3
None to probable	4
None to definite	0
Possible to definite	0
Insufficient information	9
Total	331

Source: Cobb, unpublished.

The pattern of progression shown in Table 3.6 has a special meaning with regard to the issue raised in sections 3.1 and 3.6. If nodule-forming, erosive, seropositive rheumatoid arthritis is an entity quite separate from the "polyarthritis" of the Third International Symposium, it would be reasonable to suppose that one would not precede the other. The evidence here suggests that each man climbs rather slowly through the various levels of the severity gradient and only a few reach maximum severity. Of the 17 men finally classed as definite, only three met the criteria at the first examination. On the other hand, 12 started without diagnosable rheumatoid disease or only possible disease and progressed stepwise up the ladder. While these cases of definite disease could not be called severe and most of them were serologically and radiologically negative, I see no reason to believe that the more severe cases do not move up the same severity gradient in the same way.

With this pattern of "progression" in mind it is not surprising that as the months went by increasing numbers of persons met the criteria for probable and/or definite disease. The shapes of the cumulative curves are shown in Figure 3.2. These curves rise to 5 percent for definite disease and to 14 percent for probable plus definite. Their slopes can hardly represent incidence rates, for if they did everyone in the world would soon have rheumatoid arthritis. Rather it seems that this phenomenon represents successive discovery of persons who have intermittent episodes of disease and are missed when they are examined during a remission. For example, a person who is in episode only 10 percent of the time has only a 10 percent chance of being identified at a single examination.

This kind of thinking led to the concept of describing populations by their proteps or frequency distributions according to proportion of time in episode (Beall and Cobb, 1961; Cobb, 1962). This method, although elegant, requires repeated examination of the samples, that is, at least two examinations three months apart. However, using this technique it has been possible to extend the fact that the point prevalence of pain on motion or tenderness is greater in men over 45 than it is in men under 45 (see Figure 3.3). The new information reveals that the difference is largely a result of the older men spending a larger proportion of their time in episode rather than a greater number of persons being affected. This technique deserves to be used in intergroup comparisons applied to rheumatoid arthritis, not just pain on motion or tenderness.

Longitudinal studies of population groups are of great importance

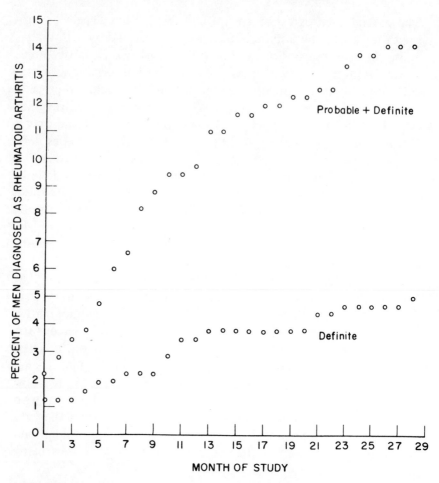

Fig. 3.2 Cumulated frequency of persons diagnosed rheumatoid arthritis, Oak Ridge (Tennessee), September 1957 through December 1960. (Reproduced with permission from Lincoln and Cobb, 1963.)

not only because they make protep estimation possible, but also because they will reveal much that now remains hidden about the natural history of rheumatoid disease. Before leaving this topic, let us examine the problem introduced by observer variation. It is always important to minimize observer variation by training the observers and by using multiple observers, as discussed above in sections 3.2–3.4. This was done in the studies of employed men referred to above. Specifically, no man was accepted as meeting the criteria for probable or definite rheumatoid arthritis unless two and usually three observers agreed that the criteria had been met. If there was disagreement

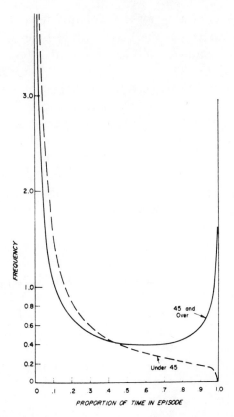

Fig. 3.3 Frequency distribution of men according to the proportion of time spent with observable evidence of pain on motion or tenderness in their joints. Men under 45 compared with men 45 and over. (Reproduced with permission from Cobb, 1962.)

between observers, the man's classification was not changed without further observation.

Even when errors have been minimized in this way, there is a tendency for the errors to accumulate because the rule "once a rheumatoid, always a rheumatoid" acts as a one-way filter. It causes cumulated prevalence rates to be overestimates of the truth without any bias toward overreporting on the part of the observers. By contrast, there is no such built-in bias in the frequency distribution according to proportion of time in episode, or protep. That is, if the observer neither over nor underreports, reasonable errors will not seriously bias the protep. However, it is my impression that a high frequency of random error will tend to bias the shape of the curve toward a low proportion of time in episode. Systematic observer bias will of course influence the area under the curve, but intuitively it would seem likely that the biases would have to be unreasonably large before they would introduce significant differences in the shapes of the distributions. This whole matter of the effects of observer error on the protep deserves careful mathematical investigation.

The possibility that the data from this longitudinal study might be so heavily contaminated with observer variation as to be meaningless has been considered. First, it has been reported (Beall and Cobb, 1961) that there is quite good agreement between the protep for joint swelling based on periodic self-report and that based on periodic examination. Second, the frequency distribution of observed episodes of swelling does not fit a Poisson distribution, X^2 with three degrees of freedom equals 170. Third, the distribution of length of reported first episodes of swelling does not fit a probability model. Fourth, the observed manifestations have prognostic value, which they would not have if they were simply random variations of the observer.

The evidence on the fourth point is presented in Table 3.7. Here the proportion of men developing an episode that could be classified as probable or definite arthritis is related to the manifestations they display during the first four months. The column of most interest is the last, which is the difference between the two preceding columns. These numbers represent the proportion of men developing an episode that could be classified as probable or definite rheumatoid arthritis, given that in the first four months of observation they had the specified manifestations but did not meet the criteria for classification as probable or definite. It should be noted that observations in the first four months are methodologically entirely independent of the subsequent classification. It is therefore truly prognostic to state that a man who was observed with pain on motion or tenderness on two occasions in four months was nine times as likely to acquire a diagnosis of rheumatoid arthritis in the next two years as was a man on whom no such observation was made.

Table 3.7 has useful implications for the selection of diagnostic criteria. It is hoped that as further longitudinal studies are developed, more analyses of this nature will be presented.

3.10 Medical Care and Disability. Given the amount of survey attention that rheumatoid disease has received, it seems quite remarkable that there is such a dearth of information about treatment, hospitalization, and disability. Perhaps it is well to start by observing that appreciable numbers of people with readily diagnosable rheumatoid arthritis are not under medical care. Kellgren and his associates

Table 3.7 The proportion of men meeting the diagnostic criteria for
probable rheumatoid arthritis by the end of the fourth month
and by the end of the twenty-eighth month given the specified
observations during the first four months of the observation
period

Diagnostic criteria observed in the first 4 months	No.	Proportion of men meeting the criteria for probable or definite rheumatoid arthritis		
		By 4 mos.	By 28 mos.	Between 4 and 28 mos.
Pain on motion or tenderness				
Observed two or more times	85	0.11	0.39	0.28
Observed once	57	0.02	0.14	0.12
Not observed	171	---	0.03	0.03
Morning stiffness for at least 30 minutes				
Reported two or more times	34	0.24	0.59	0.35
Reported once	30	0.07	0.23	0.16
Not observed	249	0.00	0.09	0.09
History of swelling				
Reported two or more times	24	0.38	0.71	0.33
Reported once	23	0.04	0.22	0.18
Not reported	266	0.00	0.09	0.09
Total	313	0.04	0.15	0.11

Source: Unpublished data from the Pittsburgh Arthritis Study.

(1953) report that about 20 percent of men and 40 percent of women
with the disease have not seen a doctor for five or more years. In the
employed population studied at Oak Ridge, only a little over half the
men with rheumatoid arthritis had ever seen a doctor about this
disease and appreciably less than half had seen a doctor in the past
year about their arthritis. Furthermore, there was a strong relationship between the number of physician visits per year and the proportion of time in episode with joint swelling (Beall and Cobb, 1961).

Figures on the number of persons treated for rheumatoid arthritis
at some time during the year from the Health Insurance Plan of
Greater New York (Densen, 1956) turn out to be 3.0 per 1,000 for
persons 15 years of age and over. This is only a small fraction of the
roughly 3 percent of persons in this age group found to have the
disease in surveys in the United States (Cobb *et al.*, 1957*b*; Mikkelsen
et al., 1963; National Center for Health Statistics, 1966*c*).

The lack of correspondence between these two kinds of data is probably caused partially by social-desirability affects leading patients to overreport the extent and recency of their medical care, and partially by a bias toward young families as numbers of HIP. However this may be, the fact remains that a sizable proportion of people with diagnosable rheumatoid arthritis are not receiving any medical supervision. This means that surveys using physicians as sources of information will substantially underestimate the frequency of the disease.

Furthermore, if one assumes that persons with diagnosable rheumatoid arthritis should have their status reviewed by a physician at least once a year, then it is reasonable to estimate that something over half of the 2,500,000 rheumatoids in the United States are receiving inadequate medical care.

I have been unable to find any useful data for the United States giving disability specific to rheumatoid arthritis. True, Brown and Lingg (1961) tell us that the employee with rheumatoid arthritis working for the Consolidated Edison Company of New York who consults the industrial physician about his condition loses an average of ten days per year because of his disease. Unfortunately, it does not seem appropriate to generalize from this small and rather special experience. It would be a real advance if we could have the kind of data presented in Chapter 2 broken down by diagnosis.

Some data of this sort are available from Great Britain (Ministry of Health, 1924; Stocks, 1948). The first of these reports is based on an insured population of 90,891 persons and the days of sick benefits per year are given by age and sex. When these specific rates are applied to the population interviewed by Stocks, one gets an estimated number of days lost that is about ten times as high as the figure determined by Stocks. One must therefore conclude that interview methods are inadequate to our purpose and that what is needed are more, and more recent, diagnosis-specific data on insured populations giving morbidity and medical-care statistics. Since the Ministry of Health data remain the best available, they are presented in Figure 3.4.

More recently, data on number of consultations and number of persons consulting a physician for rheumatoid arthritis have been provided for Great Britain by Logan and Cushion (1958). The relevant data are presented in Table 3.8.

3.11 Mortality. It has been adequately demonstrated that deaths among those who have severe rheumatoid arthritis occur at a some-

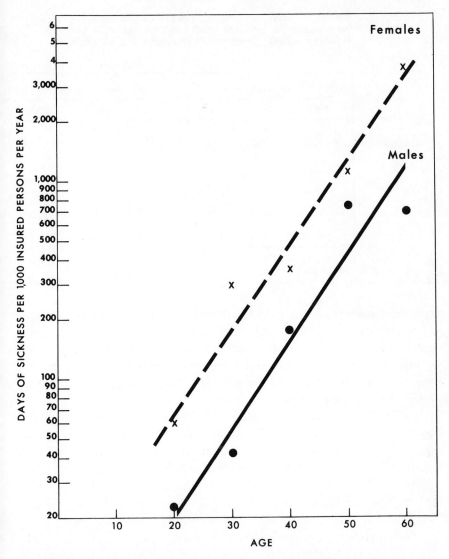

Fig. 3.4 Days of sickness attributed to rheumatoid arthritis per 1,000 insured persons per year. (Ministry of Health of Great Britain, 1924.)

what higher rate than among the rest of the population of similar age and sex (Cobb *et al.*, 1953; van Dam *et al.*, 1961; Duthie *et al.*, 1964). The excess mortality is more striking among those under age 50, but even in this group mortality is hardly an important feature of the disease.

Among the Pima Indians, excess mortality seems to be associated more with a positive serologic test than with rheumatoid disease

Table 3.8   Number of consultations and number of patients consulting
for rheumatoid arthritis per 1,000 persons per year for
selected general practices in England and Wales, 1955

Age	Consultations			Patients consulting		
	Total	Male	Female	Total	Male	Female
All ages	36.2	17.6	52.7	4.8	2.0	7.3
0-14	0.3	0.2	0.4	0.1	0.0	0.1
15-44	10.3	3.6	16.2	1.6	0.6	2.4
45-64	67.8	36.9	94.8	8.9	4.1	13.1
65 +	114.9	61.8	150.3	14.5	6.3	19.9

Source: Logan and Cushion, 1958.

(Bennett and Burch, 1968*b*). The causes of this excess mortality appear to be peptic ulcer, infection, and amyloid disease. In addition, there appear to be small excesses of deaths arising from cervical cord compression from atlanto-axial dislocation and pulmonary embolism, presumably caused by the inactive life of the cripple (Cobb *et al.,* 1953; Ball, 1968).

In Ball's study there was also a striking excess of deaths attributed to periarteritis. The possibility that this excess of periarteritis, like the excess of peptic ulcer and infection, may partially result from prolonged steriod administration must be taken into account. However, as will be noted later (section 4.8), there is an association of rheumatoid arthritis with peptic ulcer and with infection even in groups to which steroids have not been administered.

The mortality attributed to rheumatoid disease in the United States is only 6.8 per million. The rates increase with age and are higher for women than for men, as will be shown in Table 7.1. However, in only 15 percent of the death certificates in which rheumatoid arthritis is mentioned is it given as the underlying cause (Dorn and Moriyama, 1964). Furthermore, death certificates even after an autopsy usually fail to reflect the clinical diagnosis of rheumatoid arthritis. In 55 percent of a series of eighty known rheumatoids whose death certificates were examined by Atwater and Jacox (1967), no evidence suggesting arthritis could be found on the death certificate. Of course, in some of these the arthritis may not have contributed to the death even though it was a condition of long standing. Caution is therefore imperative in the interpretation of mortality data. Despite the risks we shall, in the next chapter, make the assumption that deaths attributed to rheumatoid arthritis are an unbiased sample of all deaths of persons with severe rheumatoid disease; on the basis of this assumption we shall compare and contrast the results of morbidity and mortality studies.

3.12 Overview. The point prevalence of rheumatoid arthritis is about 3 percent for the age group 35 to 64. With repeated observations on the same population additional cases in persons who are only occasionally in episode are uncovered. The true frequency of persons who have had an episode meeting the criteria of the American Rheumatism Association for probable rheumatoid arthritis must be in excess of 15 percent. At the other end of the spectrum, those who are crippled by the disease are relatively few and those who die of it constitute only 6.8 per million.

4 / THE EPIDEMIOLOGY OF RHEUMATOID DISEASE

4.0 Introduction. Having seen something of the problems of classification and having estimated the frequency of various aspects of rheumatoid disease, we are now ready for a look at specific variables and how they affect the frequency of this disease.

4.1 Age and Sex. There is general agreement that rheumatoid disease increases in frequency with age and that the moderate form of the disease is more common in women than it is in men. This pattern of increase with age, and more in females than males, is common to essentially all the studies that have been reported. The age-sex specific prevalence rates for probable, definite, and classical rheumatoid arthritis are depicted in Figure 4.1. The logarithmic relationship of age to prevalence is common but by no means universal.

Much less widely recognized is the phenomenon that appears in Table 4.1. Here it is shown that only for the rubric of definite rheumatoid arthritis is there a substantial excess of females over males. In the other rubrics, both those that suggest less severe disease and those that suggest more severe disease, the excess is relatively trivial. Somewhat similar findings have resulted from a number of other studies (Cobb *et al.*, 1957*a*; Ball and Lawrence, 1961; Lawrence *et al.*, 1961; Adler *et al.*, 1967 *a* and *b*; Mikkelsen *et al.*, 1967; Wood, 1968). In many of these studies, the bulk of the excess of moderate rheumatoid arthritis in women comes in the age group 40 to 59. I believe that this is an epidemiologic point that must be taken into account in the understanding of the disease even though the findings are not completely uniform. Wood (1968) points out that it is primarily clinical polyarthritis that is excessively frequent among women. Masi (1967) has called attention to the fact that in some surveys the rates do not rise continuously as depicted in Figure 4.1 but have a tendency to fall off in later years.

The reason for this occasional decline in prevalence in the later years is not clear. In many instances the number examined in the older age groups is small so that the estimates are quite unreliable. In some surveys the decline may result from biased sampling of older people (for example, neglecting those in institutions for chronic care), or to response bias (such as older people with arthritis refusing examination). One might postulate an effect of selective mortality, but the

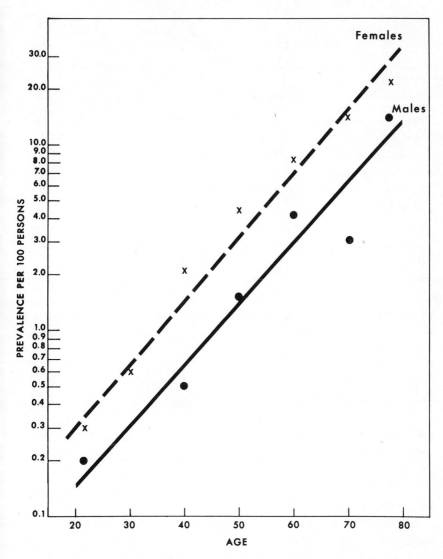

Fig. 4.1 Prevalence of probable rheumatoid arthritis in the continental United States by age. (National Center for Health Statistics, 1966b.)

excess mortality is not sufficient to produce such large changes unless one also postulates that the incidence of new cases dropped to nearly zero at some specified age. Finally, one must consider the possibility that the drop may simply be caused by cohort effects (Case, 1956). If this were so, one would posit that in those populations in which the rates level off in the older age groups there might be a tendency

Table 4.1   The frequency per 100 persons of various degrees of severity of rheumatoid arthritis and of certain manifestations of the disease by sex, with sex ratios

Manifestation or Severity	Males	Females	M/F
Morning stiffness	13.1	16.5	0.8
Swelling in only one joint	1.7	1.8	0.9
Probable rheumatoid arthritis	2.3	3.3	0.7
Definite rheumatoid arthritis	0.3	1.2	0.2
Classical rheumatoid arthritis	0.2	0.2	1.0
Positive BFT	3.4	3.5	1.0
Positive X-ray	1.0	0.6	1.7

Source: National Center for Health Statistics, 1966ᴀ.

to more disease in the more recent cohorts, which will be carried into the older ages as time passes. This is an appropriate area for further epidemiologic investigation.

4.2 Time and Place. Rheumatoid arthritis is not a new disease. May (1897) described an Egyptian mummy dated about 2600 B.C., which he claimed was the body of a rheumatoid. Although some have disputed his conclusion, I find the description of the cervical involvement, the tempero-mandibular involvement, and the involvement of the small joints of the hands quite convincing. In my view, the "claw-hand" deformity is an indication of an additional disease which should not rule out a positive diagnosis of rheumatoid arthritis.

Eve (1890) described a case of extensive involvement of the knees dated about 1300 B.C. This might have been rheumatoid in nature. Since Eve did not describe the spine, the possibility that this was a case of ankylosing spondylitis with peripheral involvement cannot be excluded. This is an important issue because Ruffer (1921) made it clear that spondylitis was extraordinarily common in the early Egyptian mummies. However, Ruffer has described the spine of a Coptic man found at Antinoë dating from about 500 A.D. The involvement with arthritis was almost entirely limited to the cervical region; the pelvis, presumably including the sacroiliac joints, was said to be normal. This description seems to fit better with peripheral disease than with spondylitis.

In an additional case, Ruffer described the peripheral joint lesions as substantially more severe than the spinal involvement. Furthermore, he pointed out more than once that quite a number of small bones with lesions resembling peripheral rheumatoid arthritis were found, but that because of the great frequency of spondylitis and the mixing of bones in common graves it was usually impossible to tell whether the small bones showing peripheral involvement belonged to the skeletons showing spinal involvement or to others. In the face of this evidence, I find it hard to believe that rheumatoid arthritis did not exist in ancient Egypt. Nevertheless, a properly conservative approach would lead to the Scotch verdict of "not proven."

In the fifteenth century Botticelli depicted hands suggesting rheumatoid arthritis in at least one of his paintings, "Portrait of a Boy" (National Gallery, Washington, D.C.). The first acceptable clinical description of the disease, by Thomas Sydenham, appeared in 1676.

As far as geography is concerned, I know of no part of the world in which this disease has been sought by competent diagnosticians and found entirely absent, except perhaps the small island of Tristan da Cunha (Black *et al.,* 1963). Between those areas where point-prevalence surveys have been made, there are some differences that are probably meaningful. Such data as are available and seem reasonably comparable are presented in Table 4.2.

Because the disease is relatively rare below age 35, the estimates in the younger age groups are really quite unstable in the sample sizes used in the surveys. Therefore the data below age 35 are omitted. As explained in the previous section and as is evident in the table, the relationship between the prevalence in the age groups 35 to 64 and 65 and over is variable, so the latter group has been omitted from the comparison also. Even with this restricted age range there are substantial differences in age distribution of the various populations. The best single comparison is made on the basis of age-adjusted rates for the age group 35 to 64, presented in the last column of figures in the table.

When one looks at these data with a full realization of the variations in technique from one study to another and the problems of classification within one study (Gofton *et al.,* 1964), one is tempted to believe that the bulk of the difference is simply technical and sampling variation. There are, however, some points that deserve comment. First, Adler and his colleagues (1967a) have made a good case for the prevalence being lower in Israel than in most other places surveyed. Second, Lawrence and his co-workers have presented

Table 4.2   The point prevalence of rheumatoid arthritis (A.R.A. probable plus definite) in various surveys, rates per 100 persons of specified age and sex

Population	Sample Size	35-44 M	35-44 F	45-54 M	45-54 F	55-64 M	55-64 F	65+ M	65+ F	Age-adjusted rates for 35-64[b] M	Age-adjusted rates for 35-64[b] F	Source
Pittsburgh, Pa.	478[a]	0.8	1.7	0.3	7.9	1.2	7.3	0.7	14.9	0.7	5.2	Cobb, unpublished
Oak Ridge, Tenn.	331	0.9	---	3.6	---	4.2	---	---	---	2.6	---	Cobb, unpublished
Framingham, Mass.	3694	2.4	3.0	0.5	4.4	1.3	6.3	0.6	6.2	1.5	4.3	Hall, 1963
Tecumseh, Mich.	2943	0.7	1.8	1.3	4.2	0.8	8.3	2.4	8.0	0.9	4.2	Dodge, 1964
United States	4306	0.5	2.1	1.5	4.4	4.2	8.3	5.6	15.9	1.7	4.4	Nat.Cent.Hlth.Stat.,1966c
Blackfeet Indians, U.S.A	936	2.4	2.1	4.9	6.7	6.0	8.0	4.3	5.1	4.1	5.1	O'Brien et al., 1967
Pima Indians, U.S.A.	827	3.4	4.7	7.4	3.2	5.4	12.4	5.0	9.4	5.3	6.0	O'Brien et al., 1967
Haida Indians, Canada	212	-	3.3	3.0	3.7	3.7	5.5	11.0	5.0	1.9	4.0	Cofton et al., 1964
Puerto Rico	2442[c]	-	1.4	0.4	2.9	0.6	3.0	0.6	1.9	0.3	2.3	Mendez-Bryan, 1963
Jamaica Negroes	529	5.5	7.6	4.8	18.1	12.6	17.4	---	---	7.0	13.5	Lawrence et al., 1966c
Leigh and Wensleydale, GB	2234	1.1	1.9	3.4	4.0	4.9	14.5	4.1	16.0	2.8	5.6	Lawrence, 1961a
Rhonda, GB	695	0.6	---	1.7	---	5.6	9.2	---	---	2.2	---	Lawrence, 1965b
Glamorgan, GB	175	-	3.3	---	---	-	8.1	---	---	---	---	de Graaff et al., 1963
Watford, GB	258	-	-	-	2.4	3.1	12.5	4.5	8.6	0.7	5.2	Ansell and Lawrence,1965
Marken, The Netherlands	597	-	-	---	8.6	1.6	6.3	2.5	7.1	0.4	4.5	Steiner et al., 1968
Rotterdam, The Netherlands	275	---	---	---	---	3.4	12.6	---	---	---	---	de Graaff et al., 1963
Heinola, Finland	346	---	---	---	---	1.2	4.8	-	---	---	---	de Graaff et al., 1963
Heinola, Finland	358	2.4	7.4	---	15.4	-	6.1	---	17.8	1.0	9.9	Laine, 1964
Piestany, Czechoslovakia	922	-	0.8	0.8	0.8	2.8	4.2	1.3	0.9	1.0	1.6	Sitaj and Šebo, 1968
Jerusalem, Israel	524[a]	0.6	1.5	1.5	4.3	-	2.0	1.7	9.5	0.8	2.6	Adler et al., 1967a
Osaka, Japan	1997	-	0.6	-	1.2	0.5	0.6	-	2.4	0.1	0.8	Shichikawa et al., 1966

[a] Stratified sample. The number represents those examined.

[b] Adjusted to U.S. population of 1940.

[c] Number screened. Only screen-positive cases were examined.

a persuasive argument for the prevalence in Jamaicans being greater than that in American Indians, and that in American Indians being greater than that in northern Europeans. Since Lawrence has participated to some extent in all the surveys involved, this seems to be a well-reasoned conclusion.

Important side issues not noted in this table include the clear excess of rheumatoid factor in the Pima Indians (Bennett and Burch, 1968a) and a distinct excess of mild erosive arthritis in the Jamaicans (Lawrence et al., 1966b). These are phenomena that are sufficiently unusual to warrant further intensive study. Latitude has not been shown to have a clearly meaningful relationship to this disease (Lawrence et al., 1966c; Lawrence, 1968a; Burch, 1968). Barlow (1968) has suggested that the relationship to latitude may be stronger for definite than for definite plus probable disease.

Additional data on Japan not included in the table (Oshima, 1960; Wood et al., 1967) suggest that Japan may be less afflicted with this malady than other parts of the world. However, there is some reason to believe that the Japanese studies have not been as inclusive in their use of the ARA criteria as have the western studies. Similarly, Puerto Rico would seem to have less disease, but it is important to note that in the Puerto Rican study no examinations were made of those who screened negative, so one feels that those estimates must err on the low side.

Method alone can hardly account for the very large difference between Puerto Rico and Jamaica. It seems likely that intensive epidemiologic study of the Caribbean Islands might uncover differences that would lead to etiologic hypotheses. Also, Jamaica seems like a good place to do longitudinal studies of persons with mild intermittent disease in order to identify factors associated with exacerbations and remissions.

Finally, it is appropriate that studies in northern Europe be focused on severe erosive, seropositive disease because more of it is found there than in the general population of the United States (Cobb and Lawrence, 1957).

We should not overlook three within-country differences, each of which deserves further study. First, Adler and his associates (1967a) suggest that Jews living in Israel but born in Europe may have higher rates, particularly for severe disease, than those born in Africa and Asia. Second, mortality data suggest an excess of the disease in the U.S. Mountain states (Burch, 1968) (see also Table 7.2). Third,

Bachman (1963) on the basis of a physician survey has suggested that there may be substantial differences between various sections of the state of Oregon.

4.3 Race. Until recently, no data have been available with which to make racial or ethnic comparisons within populations. Now from the National Center for Health Statistics and from the work of O'Brien and his associates (1967), we have figures on several minority groups in the United States. These are presented in Table 4.3, where one can readily see that there is more rheumatoid arthritis in each of the minority groups than there is in the majority group of Caucasians.

These data appear to be in conflict with the original report of the National Health Examination Survey, which indicated no difference between Caucasians and Negroes. The difference lies in taking here the age group 35 to 64 rather than all ages as used by those reporting on the National Survey. For Negroes the rates do not increase after age 65, whereas for whites they increase sharply. As indicated above, the great variability in the shape of the age curve after age 65 is not well understood and arises in part from the unreliability of estimates, so I have elected to make all comparisons on the basis of the age group 35 to 64. Ideally this comparison should be controlled on socioeconomic status because (as will be discussed below) the lower the socioeconomic status the higher the prevalence. The available data unfortunately do not make such analyses possible.

Table 4.3   The point prevalence of rheumatoid arthritis (A.R.A. probable and definite) per 100 United States residents age 35-64 by race, age adjusted to the U.S. population of 1940

Race	Number of persons examined		Rates per 100	
	M	F	M	F
Caucasians[a]	1,436	1,663	1.4	4.1
Negro[a]	202	246	2.1	5.8
Blackfeet Indians[b]	425	338	4.1	5.1
Pima Indians[b]	304	339	5.3	6.0

[a] National Center for Health Statistics.

[b] O'Brien et al., 1967.

At this point it is appropriate to point out that the mortality data presented by Burch (1968) show higher rates for Caucasians than for Negroes. This seems paradoxical but is probably explained by the fact that the disease may be less severe in the Negro. No classical cases were observed among Negroes in the National Health Survey, where at least one would have been expected in a sample of this size. Furthermore, it was observed in the Jamaica study (Lawrence *et al.*, 1966*b*) that rheumatoid arthritis was common but mild in that population of Negroes. A further possible explanation of the paradox lies in the difference in medical care received by the several racial groups. On the one hand, the greater availability of expensive therapy for the Caucasians probably leads to more frequent use of steroids and thus to higher case-fatality rates. On the other hand, the reduced medical care available to the minority groups probably reduces the proportion of those dying with rheumatoid disease for whom the fact of their disease is recorded on the death certificate. Together these circumstances probably account for the seeming contradiction between the morbidity and the mortality data.

A few years ago (Cobb, 1965*a*) the prediction was made that the resentment engendered by minority status would contribute to an excess of rheumatoid arthritis in Negroes. Table 4.3 supports this point of view but is subject to the criticism that the observed effect may result primarily from socioeconomic status. With this in mind, a further hypothesis has been examined. If it is minority status working through resentment rather than socioeconomic status that produces the racial differences, one would expect the Caucasian-Negro differences to be larger in the urban areas where the daily contacts arouse more prejudicial behavior than in the rural areas where communications and contacts between the races are fewer.

Table 4.4 was generated to test this hypothesis, and gives it substantial support. Not only are the differences between Caucasians and Negroes larger and in the predicted direction in the urban areas, but they are slightly in the opposite direction in the rural areas; furthermore, this pattern is consistent for the two sexes. This should by no means be considered proof of the resentment hypothesis, but it seems reasonable to conclude that it is a matter deserving attention in future studies. Such studies should be controlled on socioeconomic status for the reasons to be explained below.

4.4 Family Structure. Certain family variables have been examined on more than one occasion and deserve brief attention. In 1960 Chen and Cobb called attention to a possible association of rheumatoid

Table 4.4 Point prevalence rates per 100 persons for rheumatoid arthritis in United States residents aged 35-64 by sex, race and place of residence, age adjusted to the U.S. population of 1940

Sex and race	Place of residence		
	Overall	Urban	Rural
Males			
Caucasian	1.4	1.7	1.3
Negro	2.1	2.7	0.6
Females			
Caucasian	4.1	3.8	4.9
Negro	5.8	7.0	2.7

Source: National Center for Health Statistics, 1968.

arthritis and size of sibship. Since then Francis and Epstein (1965) have observed the same in the Tecumseh study, and Bennett and Burch (1968a) have found modest support for the observation in their Indian populations, the most striking relationship being seen among the older Pima Indians. A trend in the same direction has been observed by Lawrence (1968b). The proper interpretation of this finding is not clear, but it does suggest an environmental influence taking place early in life. The related phenomenon of position in the sibship has not been shown to have any relationship to the disease (Chen and Cobb, 1960).

The relationship to marital status is less clear. This matter has been examined in at least five studies (Cobb *et al.*, 1957b; King and Cobb, 1958; National Center for Health Statistics, 1966c; Adler *et al.*, 1967a; Burch, 1968). There is no agreement among the studies, although statistically significant findings occur in some of them. Perhaps more detailed analysis is needed. In particular, it appears important to examine the matter separately by sex and possibly by socioeconomic status. With regard to the number of children, the United States data (National Center for Health Statistics, 1966c) suggest that those women who have borne no children are at lower risk of rheumatoid arthritis than those who have borne one or more, while British data (Kay and Boch, 1965) suggest that the rheumatoid women are less fertile than the others.

4.5 Socioeconomic Status. As far back as 1933, Wyatt suggested that rheumatoid arthritis might be more common among the lower social classes. Since that time, several studies have examined one or another aspect of socioeconomic status. First, let us look at income. King and Cobb (1958) and more recently the National Center for Health Statistics (1966c) have adduced evidence that men in the very lowest income brackets have excessive rates for this disease. This relationship for women is trivial — if in fact it exists at all.

From the same two sources plus Cobb and Kasl (1966), we find evidence that the disease is excessively frequent among those of lesser education. Again, this seems more striking for males than for females.

With regard to occupation, the data are not so clear. Short and his associates in 1957 reviewed the literature on the subject and came to no definite conclusion. Since then de Graaff (1962) has also failed to find a relationship. However, the National Center for Health Statistics (1966c) reports that private household and service workers of both sexes have higher rates than persons in other occupations, while those working in professional, technical, and managerial jobs have the lowest rates. Again the differences are much larger for men than for women.

It seems fair to conclude that socioeconomic status is negatively related to rheumatoid arthritis, particularly among men, and that education so far has provided the strongest and most consistent associations.

4.6 Season. It is well known that a substantial proportion of persons with rheumatoid disease have increased discomfort associated with the arrival of bad weather. By the same token, symptoms of the disease are more frequent and exacerbations more common between the beginning of October and the end of March than they are during the rest of the year (Edström, 1944; Lewis-Faning, 1950; Short *et al.,* 1957; Lawrence, 1965a; Valkenburg, 1968). This observation would support the notion that miscellaneous infections may contribute to exacerbations. It is certainly a matter to be considered in epidemiologic work, for Valkenburg (1968) suggest at least twofold differences in prevalence between the highest and the lowest months. Stated in protep language, those who are infrequently in episode are more likely to be discovered in winter than in summer.

4.7 Heredity. There are a number of recent reviews of the literature on the genetic aspects of rheumatoid disease (Blumberg, 1960;

Bywaters, 1963; Masi and Shulman, 1965; Lawrence, 1967; O'Brien, 1967; Jacox *et al.,* 1968). While there is some disagreement, the gist of the matter seems to be that the best-designed studies have found the least amount of evidence for familial clustering of the disease as a whole.

There does appear to be appreciable clustering of the severe erosive and/or seropositive disease, and the rheumatoid factor itself seems to show some familial aggregation (Lawrence and Ball, 1958; Ziff *et al.,* 1958; Ball and Lawrence, 1961). The pattern of such clustering as can be demonstrated does not suggest any clear-cut genetic mechanism. Although multiple gene transmission has not been ruled out, environmental transmission has been suggested (Schmid and Slatis, 1961; Lawrence, 1967; Bennett and Burch, 1968c). Some of the factors that may account for the earlier overemphasis on this matter have been discussed by Schull and Cobb (1969). The finding of Wood and his co-workers (1967) that there is an association of rheumatoid arthritis with blood type AB warrants further investigation since the blood types are genetically determined.

It should be noted that in recent work attention has consistently been directed to rheumatoid arthritis by itself. The possibility that there may be a genetic predisposition to acquire any of several arthritic diseases has been rather overlooked. It was Garrod (1890) who called attention to the fact that in his father's series of 500 patients with rheumatoid arthritis, a family history of the disease was obtained in only 16.8 percent; still, no fewer than 43.2 percent claimed some form of arthritis, including gout, in their families. He further reported the clinical impression that rheumatoid arthritis affects the female members of gouty families with undue frequency.

More recently, Holsti and Rantasalo (1936), Holsti and Huuskonen (1938), Edström (1941), Hartmann *et al.* (1963), and Behrend (1963) have suggested that both rheumatic fever and rheumatoid arthritis may be found in the same families. By the same token, patients with Sjøgren's syndrome (Burch *et al.,* 1963) and lupus (Morteo *et al.,* 1961; Bywaters, 1963; Ansell and Lawrence, 1963; Siegel *et al.,* 1965) appear to cluster in families with rheumatoid arthritis.

It may be that in the search for very specific genetic relationships, a general susceptibility to several diseases has been overlooked. This appears to be a promising area for further research.

4.8 Association with Other Diseases. Rheumatoid disease is both positively and negatively associated with other diseases. The clinical and pathological literature on this subject is very extensive and has never been adequately reviewed. Because of the hazards of Berkson's (1946) fallacy — that is, the increased likelihood that a person with more than one disease will be in the hospital and will be autopsied if he dies — only epidemiologic and quasi-epidemiologic studies will be considered as evidence.

At the start of the discussion, I should like to call attention to the clinically recognized overlap of interrelationships between, and sometimes indistinguishability of, rheumatoid arthritis, rheumatic fever, systemic lupus erythematosus, periarteritis nodosa, progressive systemic sclerosis, polymyositis, Sjøgren's syndrome, thyroiditis, and ulcerative colitis. In each of these diseases anomalies of immune mechanisms have been suggested. For certain purposes they deserve to be investigated as a group. Already some epidemiologic attention is being given to the possibility that at least some of these diseases may have an hereditary factor in common (for example, Burch *et al.*, 1963; Siegel *et al.*, 1965).

The epidemiologic evidence for the positive association of tuberculosis and peptic ulcer with rheumatoid arthritis in males has been presented elsewhere (Cobb and Hall, 1965). Furthermore, there seems to be a negative association of this cluster of diseases with the cluster of coronary disease, hypertension, and obesity, a relationship that may not hold true for females (Epstein *et al.*, 1965). Interesting though this may be, very little of the total variance is accounted for, so our comprehension of the diseases in question is really not helped. On the other hand, the association with infectious processes generally may have considerably more meaning, in terms of both understanding and managing the disease.

4.9 Infection. No specific infectious agent has been consistently recovered from patients with rheumatoid disease, although there probably have been many fruitless searches, the results of which, like my own, have gone unpublished (Hollander *et al.*, 1962; Barnett *et al.*, 1966; Decker, 1966). Ford (1968) has reviewed the literature and found no clear evidence for a specific infectious etiology.

Short and his associates (1957) have summarized the clinical literature and added their own impression to that of the others that infection is unduly common in the period immediately prior to onset. Lewis-Faning (1950) shows a greater frequency of infection, especially tonsillitis, in the three months preceding onset. Unfortunately, all of these reports are subject to bias from the common belief among lay people that infection is relevant to arthritis. More recently, there have appeared reports of a benign polyarthritis following rubella infection. These have been summarized by Lawrence and Bennett (1960). It is not clear whether such cases become chronic. Lee and his team (1960) think they may, or at least that symptoms of "fibrositis" may persist for some time. On the other hand, the experience of Kantor and Tanner (1962) would suggest that the cases do not become chronic. Lawrence and Bennett (1960) mention arthritis following measles and infectious hepatitis, and Berglöf (1963) reports seven cases of apparently aseptic arthritis following salmonella infection. Sit'aj and his co-workers (1964) report that 38 percent of cases of "episodic benign arthritis" followed manifest upper respiratory infection.

Rather more impressive is the report of Hollander *et al.* (1962) of an epidemic of respiratory or gastrointestinal virus disease that occurred in Philadelphia in 1956-57 and was followed by polyarthritis in fourteen cases that became seropositive chronic rheumatoid arthritis in four cases. In addition, seven cases of pre-existing rheumatoid disease were exacerbated by this infection. To this experience I can add a family epidemic with essentially identical properties occurring the following year in Pittsburgh. Of the five people infected, one was a girl of 14 who for the first and only time in her life had an episode of severe hip pain lasting about three days, and another was a woman of 41 with known mild rheumatoid disease who had an exacerbation lasting about three weeks — at least two weeks beyond the end of the symptoms of the infection. In the winter of 1962, Price and his associates (1963) observed a similar epidemic in a large family of Haida Indians. In the first two of these three epidemics, unsuccessful attempts were made to isolate the infectious agent which was presumed to be a virus. Any such epidemics that occur in the future deserve intensive study.

At this point it is appropriate to call attention to two chronic infections that are associated with rheumatoid arthritis although their relationships to onset are unknown. Tuberculosis has already been mentioned, and while the possible confusion of tuberculosis and rheumatoid lung cannot be completely ruled out, the recurrence of data on this subject from a variety of clinical and epidemiologic studies suggests that in populations where both diseases are fairly common (such as Jamaica), further study might be undertaken.

Second, amebiasis has been alleged since 1925 (Barrow and Armstrong) to be unduly frequent among rheumatoids, and in fact nearly ubiquitous in the cases of rheumatoid arthritis in Oregon (Rinehart and Marcus, 1955). In view of the widespread acceptance of the amebicide chloroquine and its rleatives in the treatment of this rheumatoid disease, it is curious that this matter has not been adequately explored. Since positive tests for the rheumatoid factor are associated with a wide variety of infections, acute and chronic, as well as viral, bacterial, and protozoal, (Brooks and Cobb, 1964; Svec and Dingle, 1965), this might be looked on as another undercultivated field of investigation.

Finally, in the last dozen years there have appeared at least eight reports covering about thirty-five cases of suppurative arthritis complicating rheumatoid disease (Rimoin and Wennberg, 1966). Kellgren and his associates (1958) aptly point out that about half of the cases of suppurative arthritis admitted to the Manchester Royal Infirmary were in-patients with previously diagnosed rheumatoid arthritis. Since patients with rheumatoid arthritis form only a very small percentage of all admissions, this is certainly not a chance association. When one adds the fact that in two studies of the causes of death in rheumatoid arthritis (Cobb *et al.*, 1953; Ball, 1968) infections were excessively frequent, one is forced to the conclusion that the persons with rheumatoid disease are unusually susceptible to infection and may have a special excess of infections just prior to onset or exacerbation of disease.

4.10 Trauma. Like infection, injury, operation, and childbirth are tissue destroyers. If tissue destruction and the release of tissue antigens has a place in the etiology of rheumatoid disease, then there should be detectable association with these relevant phenomena.

All of us who have dealt clinically with rheumatoid disease are familiar with the common statement about the first joint to be involved, "Oh, I thought I had hurt it, but it hung on so long I began to wonder." Most of us have attributed this to the natural attempt to find an explanation for an affliction. However, it seems probable that these rather common statements may be fact not fiction (Kelly, 1951; Copeman, 1964). Short and his colleagues (1957) found that rheumatoid disease was reported to occur after operation, trauma, or childbirth in some 12 percent of the cases. Lewis-Faning (1950) finds a suggestive excess within one year after childbirth. Neither of the associations with childbirth are unlikely to have occurred by chance, but they are in the same direction and suggestive. There simply is not enough evidence for a conclusion pro or con.

4.11 Social Stress. There is a long list of authors who have expressed clinical opinions that emotionally significant social stresses of a wide variety are commonly associated with the onset of rheumatoid disease and/or its exacerbations. Most of these appear in the older literature and are adequately summarized elsewhere first by my father (Cobb *et al.,* 1939) and later by King (1955). Using a technique worthy of more widespread use, Cobb and his co-workers (1939) obtained medical histories and social histories quite independently on fifty patients with rheumatoid arthritis. In 62 percent of the cases a "close temporal relationship between the life stress and the arthritis" was apparent. By contrast, such a temporal relationship was found in only 12 percent of controls with varicose ulcers.

Lewis-Faning (1950) asked 292 rheumatoids and a matched control sample about seven specific social stresses preceding onset of the disease, or the equivalent date for the control, and found no difference in frequency. Unfortunately the controls in this study were largely (192 out of 302) patients hospitalized for repair of hernia or as a result of injuries. As has been noted (Kasl and Cobb, 1964; Cobb *et al.,* 1965; Carroll and Haddon, 1965), this may constitute a serious bias. In a current study of people changing jobs, there appears to be a distinct excess of mild joint swelling occurring shortly after the termination of employment. This excess was not present twelve or twenty-four months later.

Looking at the more chronic forms of social stress, we have already noted the association of low socioeconomic status and minority-group status with the disease. In the marriage area, Lewis-Faning (1950) suggests that young married males are at substantial excess risk. The other studies of civil state noted above have not been broken down by age, so there is no confirmation of this finding, which could be caused by some vagary of Lewis-Faning's study group — clearly not a random sample of patients with rheumatoid arthritis. Marital status incongruence (Kasl and Cobb, 1969*b*) and the related marital hostility (Kasl and Cobb, 1969*a*), as well as the process of getting a divorce (Cobb *et al.,* 1959) are all related to the disease. Finally, Jacox and his associates (1968), in a study of monozygotic twins discordant for rheumatoid arthritis, describe the affected twins as differing from the unaffected twins in experiencing "a series of life events which are inferred to be demanding and restricting. The quality of these life events has a tendency to be similar in the different individuals studied, and we have chosen the term entrapment to denote the particular nature of this psychological stress experience."

4.12 Personality. By personality is meant any relatively enduring psychological characteristic of the individual without reference to a particular theoretical frame. There is an extensive clinical literature relating personality to rheumatoid arthritis. This has been reviewed by King (1955), Moos (1964), Prick and van de Loo (1964), Geist (1966), and Rimón (1969). In addition, there have been a few carefully executed comparisons of rheumatoids and controls on a variety of personality dimensions using a variety of instruments. Many of these studies fail to separate men from women in the analysis. This may be of crucial importance, as will be seen below.

Taking the information garnered from the above studies and sketching the pattern with broad brush strokes, we may say that the person with rheumatoid arthritis appears oversensitive to anger and threats to self-esteem; when made angry, he is most apt to turn his anger inward. In the broadest sense of the word, he is rigid, inhibited, and sometimes described as obsessive-compulsive. Though less well confirmed with objective measure, there appears in these people an unusual vigor, or drive; and they are not infrequently described as compliant, self-sacrificing, and masochistic.

This is not the place for a full and detailed review of the evidence, so the interested reader is encouraged to seek the original sources. He will find that considering the state of the art, the agreement is surprisingly good but that relatively little of the total variance is accounted for. It is important for me to state clearly that I do not believe that personality by itself contributes anything to rheumatoid arthritis. Personality factors contribute only as they interact with specifically relevant factors in the social environment. For example, it is understandable that a subservient and rigid individual can fall into the "entrapment" of Jacox *et al.* (1968) when confronted with a difficult family situation. Further, it is easy to see how this individual who is sensitive – that is, vulnerable to anxiety, depression, and resentment – can be filled with negative affect as a result of his "entrapment" and because of his rigid, inhibited nature cannot obtain relief through overtly expressing that affect.

4.13 Early Life. There is evidence (Harburg *et al.,* 1969; Kasl and Cobb, 1969b) that women with rheumatoid arthritis come from families where there is much status stress. More specifically, these arthritic women are unduly likely to report a discrepancy between the occupational and educational levels of the father or between the educational levels of the mother and father. In these high-status-stress families the daughters report that the mother was arbitrary in her use of authority and that they resented the mother's behavior. These same daughters have more depression, more anger, and more rheumatoid arthritis.

For men, the situation seems to be reversed. There is a tendency for the male rheumatoids to come from families relatively free of status stress and to report the mother as less arbitrary and resented. This whole matter needs investigation on a larger sample of men, and with better measuring instruments.

Table 4.5 presents the key points in this area from my study of the intrafamilial transmission of rheumatoid arthritis. These are not idiosyncratic reports of maternal behavior, for they are supported by reports of siblings. However, this complex measure suffers from some of the difficulties usually attributed to multiple-regression analysis, in that subsequent studies might well not find as strong relationships. No such relationships to reports on the father were found.

To date there is no direct information on the association of these early-life factors with the personality characteristics discussed in the preceding section.

4.14 Affect and Behavior. The clinical literature abounds with comments that intrapsychic conflict over the handling of aggression is often found in persons with rheumatoid arthritis. The relevant literature has been reviewed by Cobb (1959) and Prick and van de

Table 4.5   The relationship between rheumatoid arthritis and the reporting of mother as arbitrary and resented

Sex	Mother arbitrary and resented	RA	No RA	Total
Females[a]	High score	30	20	50
	Low score	18	76	94
	All females	48	96	144
Males[b]	High score	4	87	91
	Low score	12	59	71
	All males	16	146	162

Source: Cobb and Kasl, 1968.

[a] $x^2 = 22.7$, P less than .001.

[b] Fishers exact test, P less than .01

Loo (1964). Using a scale of anger-impulsiveness in three different populations, Cobb and Kasl (1968) have shown consistent results for men and an important sex difference, as demonstrated in Table 4.6.

In this table the results are presented as standard scores, that is, the number of standard deviations away from the mean for the relevant control group. It should be noted that the women with rheumatoid arthritis are significantly more angry and impulsive than healthy women and than men with the disease. This striking difference suggests a reason for the somewhat conflicting results from earlier studies. The sex difference in the handling of anger by rheumatoids has been supported with a variety of other measures, some general and some spouse-specific (Kasl and Cobb, 1969a).

Of course, this sex difference fits with the above noted sex difference in social situations in early life. Furthermore, it predicts that married couples in which the wife has the disease should have high marital hostility, while those couples in which the husband has the disease should have low hostility. Not only is this prediction true (Kasl and Cobb, 1969a), but the further prediction that the high hostility in the families with the wife having arthritis should lead to excess peptic ulcer in the husband has also been supported (Cobb et al., 1969b).

On the other side of the coin, it is of interest that men who have acted out their aggressions, broken the law, and are being punished by imprisonment appear to have much less rheumatoid arthritis than

Table 4.6   The relation of anger impulsiveness to rheumatoid arthritis in three separate studies

Population	Males with rheumatoid arthritis		Females with rheumatoid arthritis	
	Number	Standard score	Number	Standard score
Blue collar workers in Tennessee vs. their healthy coworkers	25	-0.35	---	---
V.A. hospital patients vs. their brothers and brothers-in-law	13	-0.40	---	---
Family study cases vs. their healthy relatives	17	-0.51	49	+0.23

Source: Cobb and Kasl, 1968.

one would expect in a general population sample (Rothermich and Philips, 1963). I have personally reviewed the data from this study and recognize serious problems in the methods. First, only 4,040 prisoners were examined out of some 15,000. The 11,000 not examined were out on the farm and were more trusted; they might have been quite different from those who were examined. Second, the screening procedures used might well have led to an underestimate of the frequency in comparison with the Pittsburgh and Tecumseh studies, which are the nearest populations studied. Finally, age breakdowns of the data were not available so that age adjustments could not be performed. Despite these difficulties it is my opinion that there probably is less rheumatoid arthritis among the male prisoners kept in a high-security prison than among an equivalent age-sex group living in the community. This study deserves replication using proper survey methods.

Both men and women with rheumatoid disease score higher than controls on a variety of measures of negative affective states (Kasl and Cobb, 1969a). The association with the measures of anxiety, depression, low self-esteem, and low self-confidence are statistically significant, but, as has been pointed out by Nalven and O'Brien (1964), some of the measures contain items that are manifestations of the disease such as easy fatigue and difficulty getting started in the morning. This fact may lead to some exaggeration of the association of rheumatoid arthritis and depression.

If depression is associated with rheumatoid disease, one would expect suicide to occur with high frequency among rheumatoids. The expectation is fulfilled by the report of Dorpat and his associates (1968), who found rheumatoid arthritics several times as frequently as one would predict among those committing suicide. Of course, it is inappropriate to draw any inference about causation from a simple association of this sort, for one does not know whether the suicide results from the same cause as the rheumatoid arthritis or just from the pain of the arthritis or some combination of the two.

In summary, there is a problem about the expression of hostility here. I doubt that the men with this disease are actually less angry and resentful than the women, although they clearly neither report their anger nor express it to their wives. Elsewhere, I have reported a case illustrating this point (Cobb, 1959) and I could add others.

4.15 Negative Association with Psychosis. There are five studies of the frequency of rheumatoid arthritis among the mentally ill (Nissen and Spencer, 1936; Gregg, 1939; Trevanthan and Tatum, 1954; Pilkington, 1956; Rothermich and Philips, 1963). From a methodologic standpoint not one of these studies is comparable to the population studies that were presented in Table 4.2. In addition, I have examined the records of the Lovett Fund Study at the Massachusetts General Hospital for rheumatoid arthritics developing psychosis. From these data the following points are suggested: (a) there is no evidence for a positive or negative association of rheumatoid arthritis and mental deficiency or psychoneurosis; (b) active rheumatoid arthritis is very rare in psychotics who are out of contact, and rheumatoid arthritics become psychotic only when their arthritis is in remission; (c) the evidence is inadequate to determine whether psychosis and rheumatoid disease are negatively associated in persons, though they clearly do not appear to coexist contemporaneously.

The meaning of this lack of co-occurrence of the active phase of these two disease processes is not clear. Perhaps it should be interpreted eventually in the light of Funkenstein's (1950) observation of the alternation of psychotic and asthmatic symptoms; and in the light of the observation that visible physical defects are uncommon among mental patients (Weiss and Bergen, 1968).

4.16 A Theory. At this point, I am going to propose a theory about the genesis of rheumatoid arthritis. I do this fully recognizing that the proposed theory may be incorrect in part, or even in several parts. I do it because I believe strongly that the time has come to move away from point-prevalence estimates and on to the examination of hypotheses about the etiology of the disease. I make no claim that the theory is original. In fact, much of it has been stated by Solomon and Moos (1964). What is presented here should be looked on as an extension of and further support for the notions they integrated.

Figure 4.2 represents my present concept of the etiology of rheumatoid disease. The black box represents the area of clinical investigation. Starting at the left, we have examined the evidence for infection or trauma and for social stress being associated with onset and exacerbation. Clinical impressions are strong in these areas and modest epidemiologic evidence supports these opinions. The fact that the associations individually seem weak is not in conflict with the theory, which predicts strong relationships to the concatenation of the factors but not to the individual factors. In this connection the observation of Short and his associates (1957) is relevant: "The most com-

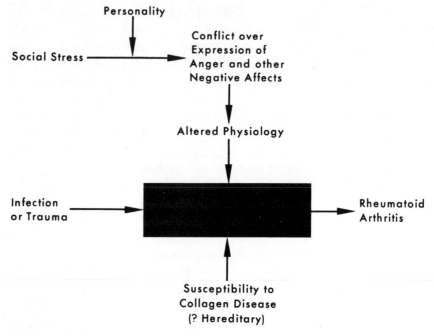

Fig. 4.2 Schematic presentation of epidemiologically derived hypotheses about the etiology of rheumatoid arthritis. The black box remains the province of clinical investigation.

mon combination was strain of long duration before an onset immediately preceded by an infection, operation or injury."

When one adds to these environmental events the special personality characteristics that make an individual vulnerable to social stress, as discussed in section 4.12, one gets a logical flow from the social stress to the conflict over expression of anger and other negative affects. It has been amply demonstrated (Mason, 1968) that negative affect is associated with physiologic changes, particularly the output of the adrenal glands. In section 4.7 attention was directed to the possibility that there may be an hereditary susceptibility to collagen disease. How these three factors get put together in the black box is a matter for clinical investigation. I believe that the clinical research task is to study exacerbations and remissions in persons with mild intermittent rheumatoid arthritis. It is only when we understand the mechanisms involved that the significance of the epidemiology will be clear.

5 / DEGENERATIVE JOINT DISEASE

5.0 Introduction. There is no clear agreement about the appropriate name for the condition that will be discussed next. The "Primer on the Rheumatic Diseases" prepared by a committee of the American Rheumatism Association (1964) prefers the term *degenerative joint disease.* From the point of view of the author, it is difficult to defend calling the condition a disease when, so far as can be determined at present, it affects all persons who live long enough. In a sense this is merely quibbling over words, but the point is made; the condition is ubiquitous. For convenience, I shall speak of osteoarthrosis as involving diarthrodial joints and distinguish it from intervertebral disk degeneration, even though it is not established that these conditions are etiologically separate.

Classification with regard to these conditions is for all practical purposes a radiological matter. According to the *Atlas of Standard Radiographs of Arthritis* (1963), the following radiological features are considered evidence of osteoarthrosis:

(a) Formation of osteophytes on the joint margins or in ligamentous attachments, as on the tibial spines;

(b) Periarticular ossicles; these are found chiefly in relation to the distal and prosimal interphalangeal joints;

(c) Narrowing of joint space associated with sclerosis of subchondral bone;

(d) Altered shape of the bone ends, particularly the head of femur.

The following radiologic features are evidence of disk degeneration: narrowing of the disk space, sclerosis of the vertebral plates, and marginal osteophytes.

5.1 Pain. From an epidemiologic standpoint pain, which is a part of osteoarthritis, is not usually associated with degenerative joint disease. That is to say that most degenerative joint disease is relatively pain free. When pain is associated it is probably due to one of the following:

(a) When osteophytes develop rapidly, there may be associated localized pain, tenderness, redness, and sometimes swelling. This process is seen most clearly in the most exposed joints, namely, the terminal interphalangeal joints of the fingers. The process here is so conspicuous that the resulting nodes have come to carry the eponym of Heberden. It is the author's untested suspicion that the process in these terminal interphalangeal joints is better described and better understood simply because of the exposed location, and it is postulated that were the hip and the knee equally visible and accessible to the palpating hand, a similar process would be recognized in these joints as well.

(b) An osteoarthrosic joint may become painful when it is "overused." In this instance the definition of overuse is, of course, the amount of use that produces pain. As the condition progresses, the amount of use that can be tolerated without pain is reduced. It is, however, important to remember that the joint affected solely by this condition should be free of pain and swelling when it is not "overused," and that some people can use osteoarthrosic joints extensively without pain. When pain and swelling do occur as a result of overuse, the joint fluid is free of signs of inflammation and the reaction disappears in a short period of time, a matter of days rather than weeks.

(c) When the spine is involved, there may be nerve-root compression caused by the thinning of the intervertebral disks and/or osteophytes which project into the intervertebral foramina.

(d) Finally, there is good reason to believe that a substantial proportion of what is commonly called "osteoarthritis" is merely mild rheumatoid arthritis of good prognosis in older people who have degenerative changes visible by X-ray. Stated another way, those who have the minimal form of rheumatoid arthritis are likely to have pain from their osteoarthrosic joints, whereas those who have no such tendency are usually more free of pain (Cobb *et al.*, 1957*a*). The separation is obviously not clean, for the swelling of overuse may merge into the swelling derived from a minimal tendency to rheumatoid disease. In my opinion soft tissue swelling and/or fluid lasting weeks rather than days is a reason for looking for an additional process beyond the osteoarthrosis visible by X-ray.

5.2 The Clinical Syndromes that come under the general rubric of osteoarthrosis seem to fall into three categories.

(a) Primary osteoarthrosis, which at the present time seems to include the bulk of the problem with which we are concerned. All joints in the body are subject to degenerative changes with varying degrees of rapidity, and therefore become evident at different ages. Certain joints such as the terminal interphalangeal joints of the fingers are conspicuously involved as noted above, and the evolution of the nodes on these joints has been well described

(Kellgren and Moore, 1952; Stecher, 1955; Jackson and Kellgren, 1957). It seems quite likely that a similar process takes place in other joints but that, because routine examination of joints at autopsy is the exception rather than the rule, the early and transient stages of this process are rarely observed. It is probable that generalized osteoarthrosis (Francon, 1950; Kellgren and Moore, 1952; Wardle, 1953) is merely the most severe form of this process, which begins with a single joint and proceeds to multiple involvement, each joint going through its evolution at its own rate.

(b) Secondary osteoarthrosis may result from trauma or from abnormal wear related to obesity or postural abnormalities; to congenital disease including alcaptonuria (La Du et al., 1958), congenital dislocation of the hip (Barrie et al., 1958), chondrodysplasia, and perhaps ligamentous laxity (Brown and Rose, 1966); and to external intoxication as in Kashin Beck's disease (Nesterov, 1964). Further, it seems likely that osteoarthrosis progresses more rapidly in the presence of rheumatoid arthritis. This is a touchy matter, because it is equally appropriate to say that these changes are a part of rheumatoid disease. It is not clear whether the erosive osteoarthritis of Crain (1961), Peter et al. (1966), and Kidd and Peter (1966) belongs in this category.

(c) Disk degeneration is usually separated from the rest of osteoarthrosis partly because of the sex differences, disk degeneration being more prevalent in males and osteoarthrosis more common in females. This differentiation is based primarily on the impression that the involvement of interfacetal joints is reasonably independent of the changes in the disks and vertebral bodies. This impression is not fully borne out by the data of Lewin (1964), from whose work have been calculated the following correlations averaged across the several lumbar segments. For osteoarthrosis of synovial joints with osteophytes on the margins of the body $r = 0.23$, for osteoarthrosis with disk narrowing $r = 0.44$, and for marginal osteophytes with disk narrowing $r = 0.44$. These correlations compare favorably with correlations found by O'Brien and his associates (1968) between DIP and MCP joints, suggesting that there may not be as important a distinction between osteoarthrosis and disk degeneration as was believed. Furthermore, Kellgren and Lawrence (1958) found significantly more disk degeneration in persons with osteoarthrosis of the distal interphalangeal joints than in those without. Clearly, some additional study of these relationships is indicated.

5.3 Observer Variation is important even in this condition which is entirely a radiological diagnosis. The total of observer variation clearly is the sum of that variation resulting from technique and that caused by the readers. One naturally assumes that the former variation is small, but so far as can be determined it has not yet been measured. On the other hand, there are substantial amounts of data on the inter- and intra-observer variation in reading the same X-rays.

Table 5.1 presents the correlations between readers and within readers over time for various joints. In each instance, five-point scales (0 to 4) were used, but of course the marginal distributions vary considerably. Since the correlation coefficient is somewhat dependent on the marginal distributions, these figures should be used primarily to indicate the order of magnitude of the agreement. The most strik-

Table 5.1   Correlation between and within observers in the assessment of osteoarthrosis in various joints and groups of joints

Joints and groups of joints	Inter-observer	Intra-observer
Distal interphalangeal[a]	0.73	0.81
Metacarpophalangeal[a]	0.66	0.88
First carpometacarpal[a]	0.78	0.81
Wrist[a]	0.10	0.62
Cervical spine[a]	0.57	0.66
Dorso-lumbar spine[a]	0.52	0.42
Hips[a]	0.40	0.75
Knees[a]	0.83	0.83
Hands[b] (mean of three observers)	0.76	0.81
Feet[b] (mean of three observers)	0.61	0.74

[a] Kellgren and Lawrence, 1957a.

[b] National Center for Health Statistics, 1966a.

ing thing is that with single readings only, one cannot expect correlations between osteoarthrosis and some variable to exceed 0.7 because the remaining 50 percent of the variance will be taken up by observer error. In order to combat this, it is important to have multiple readings of X-rays.

In Table 5.1, no data on variation with regard to readings for disk degeneration have been included because none have been made available in comparable form. However, Kellgren and Lawrence (1952) have made it quite clear that important variations occur and that multiple readings are necessary here also.

When two studies are being compared, it is important that some of the X-rays be exchanged in order to get an estimate of the relationship of one reader to the other. It is not necessary to exchange full sets of X-rays unless the populations are small or one is looking for miniscule differences.

5.4 Prevalence of Osteoarthrosis. In 1942 Bennett and his co-workers pointed out that from the pathologist's standpoint the changes of osteoarthrosis in the knee begin by age 20 and involve essentially all joint surfaces by age 60. A larger series, about 1,000 autopsies, involving many joints was reported in 1926 by Heine. For those interested in the detail available from autopsy data, these two reports are the classics.

We are, here, more concerned with the radiological and clinical findings in more randomly selected populations. Quite a number of populations have been studied but the reports are usually not presented in comparable form. Lawrence and his associates (1963) have compared six populations for frequency in the 55 to 64 year age group, and suggest there is at least a real difference in frequency and pattern between the British and the Finnish samples. What seems to be needed most at the moment is an accepted minimum set of joints and joint groups that will be reported comparably and regularly from all surveys so that direct comparisons can be made. *The Atlas of Standard Radiographs of Arthritis* (1963) was the first essential step. Now a standard format for preparing the reports should be adopted, perhaps at the next International Conference on the Epidemiology of Chronic Rheumatism.

For the present, it is suggested that a minimal set of X-rays to be taken should include hands, feet, and cervical spine. In addition, it is highly desirable to have X-rays of one knee. For reporting purposes it seems appropriate to read the joing groups (hands or feet) separately and to present the results by ten-year age groups so that the slopes of the age curves can be compared.

That there are large, significant differences in these slopes for certain groups is illustrated in Figure 5.1. The readings of the films on the Pima Indians and on the United States population were done by the same readers and in the same manner. The grade of osteo-arthrosis assigned "corresponded to the grade of the most severely affected joint of the hands (but excluding any single isolated joint where the involvement was rated at least two grades more severe than the other joints in the hand)." The earlier readings on the hands of the Eskimos was done using the same grading system and involved one of the same readers. However, it would appear that the Eskimo findings may, if anything, be a little exaggerated by reporting the grade of the worst joint and by including the wrists in the reading.

From the figure it is evident that the Pima Indians have more

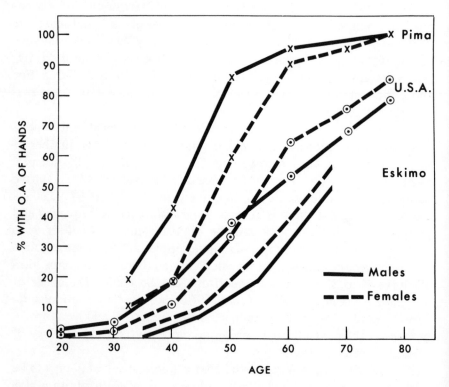

Fig. 5.1 Radiological osteoarthrosis of the hands, grades 2 to 4, by age, for three populations. (Burch, 1967; National Center for Health Statistics, 1966a; Blumberg *et al.*, 1961.)

osteoarthrosis of their hands than the rest of the U.S. population, and that the U.S. population has more disease than the Alaskan Eskimos. The sex differences are far from consistent, for the Pima males have more osteoarthrosis than their womenfolk, while the Eskimo males have less; and there is an appreciable crossover in the U.S. random sample, with the men starting higher and being over-taken by the women. This crossover appears due to an excess of mild involvement in young men and an excess of severe involvement in old women. These same patterns seem to hold for the feet, although no data are available on the feet of the Eskimos. It would, of course, be desirable to compare cervical spines and knees in a similar fashion if suitable data were available.

5.5 Prevalence of Disk Degeneration. There is little to be said on the subject of disk degeneration that was not adequately said by Lawrence and his co-workers in 1963. For the edification of the reader, their elegant figure is reproduced here as Figure 5.2. It is clear

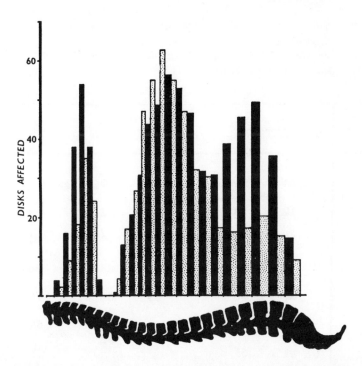

Fig. 5.2 Prevalence of grade 2 to 4 degenerative change in individual disks in random samples of 100 males and 100 females aged 35 and over. Males: black; females: stippled. (Reproduced with permission from Lawrence *et al.*, 1963.)

that there are striking differences in the frequency of the condition by site and sex. Furthermore, it increases with age, as can be seen in Table 5.2. Here the Leigh and Wensleydale data have simply been added together by the original authors.

The need for full spine films makes the epidemiology of disk degeneration somewhat cumbersome. To date, the only geographic comparisons have been of cervical involvement in the 55- to 64-year-age groups in five surveys in northern Europe. The sole impressive difference is between the sexes, with more severe degeneration in the disks of males than of females. Otherwise, it would seem to be a fair statement that about 60 percent of both males and females have some radiological evidence of this condition by the age of 60, no matter which part of northern Europe they come from.

5.6 *The Etiology* of osteoarthrosis is surely multiple, as the concept of secondary disease would imply. There are some like Collins (1953) who believe that "the inciting conditions of the disease must

5.2 The prevalence per 100 persons X-rayed of disk degeneration in the cervical, dorsal and lumbar spines of males and females from Leigh and Wensleydale, England

Age	Cervical		Dorsal [a]		Lumbar	
	M	F	M	F	M	F
15-24	1	1	13	20	---	
25-34	10	3	20	52	---	
35-44	29	20	58	79	35	21
45-54	55	51	72	83	58	39
55-64	68	68	83	86	74	53
65-74	87	74	97	92	84	68
75 +	81	65			81	79

Source: Lawrence, de Graaff and Laine, 1963.

[a] Leigh only.

be sought separately for each diseased joint." Others like Kellgren and Moore (1952) and Robecchi (1964) believe that a "primary" condition can be identified as occurring early in life, involving multiple joints with a strong hereditary tendency. In essence, the question is how much of the etiology can be attributed to wear and tear as opposed to constitutional factors. Sokoloff (1963) has reviewed the various theories in an unbiased manner and concludes that as yet we do not really know whether there are important systemic contributions to the development of the condition.

5.7 Epidemiologic Evidence for the Wear-and-Tear Theory. This theory says in essence that the longer and harder the joint is used, the more likely it is to be osteoarthrosic. In support of this theory, there is considerable epidemiologic evidence. First, the frequency of osteoarthrosis increases sharply with age; second, the lower extremities are more involved earlier in life than are the upper extremities; third, obesity is associated particularly with involvement of the lower extremities; fourth, occupational use influences the location; and fifth, poliomyelitic paralysis of a limb reduces the involvement of that limb. Each of these points will be discussed in turn.

In Figure 5.1 is seen an example of the extent to which osteoarthrosis in the hands increases with age. This is generally true for all joints in every study that has been made. So striking is the increase with age that some have felt that it was an inevitable concomitant of advancing years. Evidence will be presented below to suggest that it is the amount of use of a given joint rather than its chronologic age that influences the probability of osteoarthrosis.

In Table 5.3 are presented data from the work of Heine (1926) that indicate clearly that, both for females and males, the osteoarthrosis progresses more rapidly in the knee than in the elbow, and in the hip than in the shoulder. In order to facilitate the understanding of this table, I have calculated the ages by which 50 percent of persons have developed the condition in the relevant joint. In each instance the 50 percent point is reached earlier in the weight-bearing joints. The differences range from 15 to 19 years.

Obesity appears to contribute to the frequency of osteoarthrosis in the lower extremity but not in the upper extremity. There have been a number of clinical studies pointing this out, one of the better and more recent ones being that of Nava and Seda (1964). They found obesity in 73 percent of patients with osteoarthrosis of the lower limbs, but in only 49 percent of patients with upper-limb

Table 5.3 Percent of persons with the indicated degree of anatomical evidence of osteoarthrosis, data on 1,002 cadavers

A. The knee compared with the elbow for males and females

	Males						Females					
	Knee			Elbow			Knee			Elbow		
Age	Total	Mild	Marked	Total	Mild	Marked	Total	Mild	Marked	Total	Mild	Marked
15-19	6.7	6.7										
20-29	11.4	11.4		1.4	1.4		6.0	6.0		2.0	2.0	
30-39	62.5	62.4		30.0	30.0		38.9	37.2	1.7	10.0	10.0	
40-49	75.7	71.4	4.3	24.6	24.6		72.2	69.0	3.2	29.5	27.9	1.6
50-59	90.0	82.0	8.0	66.0	61.0	5.0	81.8	70.9	10.9	53.7	50.0	3.7
60-69	91.0	71.0	20.0	75.0	68.0	7.0	94.4	51.1	43.3	72.2	61.1	11.1
70-79	96.6	67.4	29.2	97.7	77.3	20.4	98.2	51.8	46.4	79.1	62.7	16.4
80-89	100.0	68.8	31.2	100.0	87.5	12.5	100.0	40.0	60.0	94.5	72.8	21.7
50% point	28 years			46 years			33 years			48 years		

B. The hip compared with the shoulder for males and females

	Males						Females					
	Hip			Shoulder			Hip			Shoulder		
Age	Total	Mild	Marked	Total	Mild	Marked	Total	Mild	Marked	Total	Mild	Marked
15-19												
20-29	1.4	1.4								2.0	2.0	
30-39	7.5	7.5		2.5	2.5		8.0	8.0		1.6	1.6	
40-49	17.2	12.5	4.7	2.9	2.9		16.1	14.3	1.8	6.7	5.0	1.7
50-59	46.8	38.3	8.5	13.3	9.2	4.1	39.2	39.2	-	16.0	16.0	-
60-69	57.7	47.4	10.3	27.0	14.0	13.0	61.3	49.3	12.0	16.6	10.0	6.6
70-79	66.5	44.8	21.7	50.6	28.2	22.4	76.4	50.0	26.4	39.1	20.0	19.1
80-89	71.4	64.3	7.1	40.0	6.7	33.3	82.6	50.0	32.6	65.5	40.0	25.5
50% point	53 years			70 years			55 years			74 years		

Source: Heine, 1926.

involvement. The elegant survey by Kellgren and Lawrence (1958) brings this point out particularly clearly. As shown in Table 5.4, they found that the knee joint and the metatarso-phalangeal joint of the great toe were significantly more frequently involved in obese persons than in nonobese persons and that this was true for both sexes. Their definition of obesity was 10 percent overweight by standard height-weight tables, which involved 27 percent of males and 44 percent of females.

What Kellgren and Lawrence did not say but what appears on reworking their data is that for each of the joints in the upper extremity examined, there is a small excess of osteoarthrosis among the obese. When this occurs in five consecutive joint groups, one is inclined to think on the basis of a sign test that this is not just a chance occurrence, and that the association of obesity with osteo-arthrosis may have meaning beyond the simple wear-and-tear hypothe-sis. In the central section of this table, one notes that the joints of the spine do not exhibit any clear relationship of osteoarthrosis and/or disk degeneration to obesity.

Table 5.4   The relation of obesity to osteoarthrosis in males and females combined

Joints and groups of joints	Obese		Nonobese		Obese minus nonobese
	No.	Percent with grade 2-4 changes	No.	Percent with grade 2-4 changes	
Distal interphalangeal	132	61	247	48	+13 [a]
Proximal interphalangeal	132	38	247	25	+13 [a]
Metacarpophalangeal	132	25	247	20	+ 5
Carpometacarpal	132	31	247	25	+ 6
Wrists	131	13	247	7	+ 6 [a]
Cervical spine					
Osteoarthrosis	131	25	240	24	- 1
Disk degeneration	137	68	240	63	+ 5
Lumbar spine					
Osteoarthrosis	126	36	232	24	+12 [a]
Disk degeneration	126	49	232	55	- 6
Sacroiliacs	126	6	229	10	- 4
Hips	126	17	232	14	+ 3
Knees	130	53	240	26	+27 [a]
Tarsi	132	11	247	4	+ 7 [a]
Lateral metatarsophalangeal	132	9	247	4	+ 5 [a]
First metatarsophalangeal	132	59	247	35	+24 [a]

Source: Kellgren and Lawrence, 1958.
[a] P less than 0.01

These results are confirmed by the National Center for Health Statistics (1968) although the relationship of osteoarthrosis of the hands to obesity is rather stronger for women than for men. Thus it is evident that there is substantial clinical opinion that obesity is associated with osteoarthrosis and/or the painful aspects of this condition, and that two surveys substantiate the relationship. These surveys, however, do not make completely clear whether the contribution of obesity is primarily through wear and tear or through some other mechanism. Furthermore, Kellgren (1961) points out that "obese males had nearly twice as much osteoarthrosis of the distal interphalangeal joints, and the pattern of osteoarthrosis in these males resembled that of females." Further study of this matter is clearly indicated.

Turning to occupation, we find that white-collar workers are twice as likely to apply for disability benefits for rheumatoid arthritis as for osteoarthrosis, while laborers who apply for disability have one-and-a-half times as much osteoarthrosis as rheumatoid arthritis (Roemmich, 1962). A similar conclusion was reached by Coates and Delicati (1932) in their analysis of the occupational distribution of patients admitted to the Royal Mineral Water Hospital in Bath, England. The relevant data are found in Table 5.5.

To be more specific, Kellgren and Lawrence (1952) demonstrated that coal miners have an excess of osteoarthrosis in their hands, knees, and lumbar spines; and Caplan and his fellow-workers (1966)

Table 5.5   The relative frequency of male admissions to the Royal Mineral Water Hospital in Bath, England, for osteoarthritis by type of work

Type of Occupation	Total	% Osteo-arthritis
Heavy physical labor	1517	24
Less hard outdoor and indoor occupations	619	18
Mental work with or without physical work	229	13

Source: Coates and Delicati, 1932.

showed that the degree of disk degeneration but not osteoarthrosis of the pedicle joints is related to the length and degree of heavy work in the mines. Cotton operatives (Lawrence, 1961b), like diamond cutters (Tempelaar and van Breemen, 1932) and other craftsmen (National Center for Health Statistics, 1966b), have excess osteoarthrosis in their hands. By the same token, men engaged in real estate, finance, or insurance have less (National Center for Health Statistics, 1966b). Finally, physicians seem to have a very low frequency of Heberden's nodes (Stecher, 1940).

If we look at this in quite another way, the standardized morbidity ratios for the appearance of osteoarthritis and disk disease among those receiving social-security support for disability gives striking evidence that heavy work contributes to the condition. Selected data on this subject from U.S. Department of Health, Education and Welfare (1967) are presented in Table 5.6.

Glyn and his associates (1966) derived the interesting hypothesis that persons with poliomyelitis of one leg should have less osteoarthrosis on the affected side than on the unaffected side. This proved to be strikingly true, and in fact the frequency of osteoarthrosis was not particularly different in the hips and the knees of the unaffected side from that found in normal persons. What was unusual was the very low frequency of osteoarthrosis in the hips and knees of the weaker limbs, many of which were supported by caliper braces.

A companion piece of information comes from the U.S. National Health Survey (National Center for Health Statistics, 1968), for it was shown that osteoarthrosis of the hand is related to arm girth even when corrected for skin thickness. The amount of muscle therefore is related to the extent of osteoarthrosis. This information nicely complements the observations mentioned above that joints subject to overuse caused by trauma or congenital deformity are likely to develop excessive osteoarthrosis. In this category, of course, should be included the observation by Caplan et al. (1966) that the pedicle joints in the lumbar spine are almost entirely free of osteoarthrosis unless there is disk degeneration as well, suggesting that the osteoarthrosis of these joints is secondary to the disk changes and the resulting misalignment of the joint surfaces.

In concluding this section, I must admit to being impressed with the support for the wear-and-tear hypothesis. However, I continue to feel that there must be other factors. Perhaps the relation to cholesterol level (Kellgren, 1961) and to diabetes (Waine et al., 1961) may be useful clues here, or perhaps they are only further pieces of the relation to obesity. This whole area needs additional study.

Table 5.6   Standardized morbidity ratios for osteoarthritis and
             displacement of intervertebral disk for selected light
             and heavy occupations among persons receiving United
             States social security benefits for disability

Occupation	Osteoarthritis	Displacement of intervertebral disk
Professional, technical and kindred workers	.53	.35
Managers, officials and proprietors	.50	.47
Clerical and kindred workers	.55	.55
Sales workers	.56	.59
Minerals, extraction of	1.95	2.63
Lumbermen, raftsmen and woodchoppers (skilled and semi-skilled)	2.40	1.52
Lumbermen, raftsmen and woodchoppers (unskilled)	1.91	2.08
Sawmill (unskilled)	1.95	1.13
Paper and pulp manufacture (unskilled)	1.68	2.44
Foundry (unskilled)	1.40	1.60
Petroleum (unskilled)	2.04	-
Construction (unskilled)	1.67	1.70
Longshoremen and stevedores (unskilled)	1.81	2.66

Source: U.S. Department of Health, Education and Welfare, 1967.

5.8 Heredity. As Lawrence (1960) has pointed out, there are two
ways that heredity may influence the development of osteoarthrosis.
The first is inheritance of an increased susceptibility to the wear and
tear of daily life. The second is the inheritance of factors known to
contribute to the condition either in a localized fashion, as congenital
dislocation of the hip, or in a general fashion, as in alcaptonuria. Our
concern here is with the first question as to whether there is, in fact,
a variability in the wearing qualities of the articular cartilage that is
genetically determined.

An approach to this question will require clarification of several points before sound work can be undertaken. First, clear criteria for separating primary and secondary disease are needed. The common assumption that when a single joint is involved the process is traumatic, and when multiple joints are involved it is primary or generalized, has a dangerous circularity. Second, the confusion resulting from studying clinical Heberden's nodes without X-rays that might reveal less severe grades of osteoarthrosis must be unraveled. Third, the definition of primary osteoarthrosis as that osteoarthrosis for which heredity is conspicuous (Robecchi, 1964) also has a circuitousness that leads to confusion. Finally, if the evidence of Caplan and his co-workers (1966) that osteoarthrosis of interfacetal joints in the lumbar region is found only in the presence of disk degeneration is supported, it will be apparent that osteoarthrosis of spinal interfacetal joints and disk degeneration are part of the same condition. Hopefully, this will be clarified by the across-joint correlations that are being undertaken by O'Brien and his associates (1968).

The literature on the hereditary aspects of osteoarthrosis is scattered and spotty. Rather than review it piece by piece, it seems appropriate to make a series of predictions as to what would be expected if the wear-and-tear hypothesis were combined with an hereditary difference in susceptibility to the effects of wear and tear. The following predictions suggest themselves:

(a) The distribution of persons according to number of joints involved would be bimodal or at least skewed to the high side, and this skewness would increase with the age of the sample.

(b) The difference in frequency, severity, and number of joints involved between those having a first-degree relative with osteoarthrosis and those in the general population would increase with age.

(c) These differences would also be larger in the lower extremities, particularly in obese persons, and would be magnified by occupational overuse and by deformities, both congenital and acquired.

The first point is not supported by the work of O'Brien and his fellow-workers (1968). In fact, in their data the high side of the distribution appears truncated.

Armstrong (1920), Hermann (1936), and Neri Serneri and Bartoli (1957) each demonstrated differences between those with and those without a relative having osteoarthrosis. Only Kellgren and his team (1964) took the trouble to demonstrate that the difference is more clear-cut in the older age group, thus supporting my second prediction. Stecher (1957) looked solely at Heberden's nodes, which would appear to be only a part of osteoarthrosis, and made a good case for this trait being influenced by a single autosomal gene which behaves as a dominant in the female and a recessive in the male. It is conceivable that these conclusions are not extensible to the entire condition and that what seemed to be a sex difference in the inheritance is, in fact, only a sex difference in the pattern of joint involvement.

To date, no one seems to have looked at the third point – the interaction of occupation, obesity, and deformity with the possibility of inherited susceptibility – although Robecchi (1964) has suggested that this should be important.

It seems reasonable to conclude that there is probably some hereditary contribution to an increased susceptibility of joints to osteoarthrosis, but that the mode of inheritance will not be fully worked out until the biochemical defect involved has been identified. Before concluding that there is surely a genetic influence in this situation, it is well to remember that in addition to genes, such things as property, occupational choice, and many habits are passed down in the family. This is a condition that is influenced by occupation, activity level, and obesity, so the possibility that familial habits contribute more than genetics must be considered.

5.9 Significance. Osteoarthrosis and disk degeneration are not direct causes of death, although of course they may appear on the death certificate. On the other hand, as sources of pain they are very important. They probably account for much of the reply to solicitous inquiry, which runs "Oh, I'm just getting old."

The proportion of persons with radiological osteoarthrosis who suffer from pain in the involved joints is variously estimated by different authors, depending on the severity of the joint changes and the nature of the inquiry. In general, at least 50 percent of persons with radiological osteoarthrosis do not complain of any related pain. This naturally raises the question as to whether it is possible to characterize the difference between those who have pain and those who do not.

First, both Cobb *et al.* (1957*a*) and Lawrence *et al.* (1966*a*) indicate clearly that the more severe the radiological changes, the greater the likelihood of pain. Second, the same two authors report that while osteoarthrosis is not strikingly associated with either the symptom morning stiffness or the disease rheumatoid arthritis, both markedly influence the likelihood of pain (assuming that osteoarthrosis of a specified degree is present). Third, Lawrence *et al.,* (1966*a*) have demonstrated that pain in the osteoarthrosic knee is more common among the obese than among the lean. This is in line with the clinical observation that osetoarthrosic joints are apt to become painful and even a little swollen after overuse. Fourth, Ishmael (1967) has called attention to the association of painful osteoarthrosis with migraine headaches, motion sickness, and insomnia. The suggestion that these diseases cluster in families as well as in individuals is of considerable interest. Fifth, Lawrence (1962) suggests that those exposed to cold, damp conditions are more apt to have symptoms, presumably because of the influences of tissue-cooling on the pain threshold; but a few years later Lawrence and his associates (1966*a*) were doubtful about the effect of damp housing.

Because radiological osteoarthrosis is so common in the older age groups, involving at least one joint in at least 50 percent of persons by age 50 and at least one joint in 97 percent of persons by age 65 (Lawrence *et al.,* 1966*a*), it contributes a good deal to the complaint rate and the minor-disability rate, but probably not much to serious and prolonged disability. Disk degeneration, on the other hand, may cause disability of significant duration. Neither can be considered a serious problem except perhaps in older men doing heavy work. The morbidity data in this area are far from tidy, mostly because of inadequate classification. Here again is a suitable matter for further investigation.

5.10 Overview. It appears that the degenerative joint disease results from use and abuse of joints of varying susceptibility to cartilage degeneration. A variety of specific factors have been pointed out, and it has been concluded that there may be a general, genetically determined variation in susceptibility. There are clear differences between populations in the rate of increase of osteoarthrosis with age by sex, which deserve further study. The very low rate of the condition among Alaskan Eskimos is of considerable interest.

Several kinds of field studies seem to be needed. One is a continued exploration of populations and population subgroups to identify groups that have large differences in the slope of the increase in prevalence with age. Ideally these data should be presented in detail, as in Figure 5.1. When space does not permit presentation of all the data, the use of 50 percent endpoints is appropriate, as in Table 5.3. In any case, analyses should be specific to groups of joints. I do not think that analyses simply counting the number of joints affected (such as that of Bremner *et al.* in 1968) should be repeated, for they give us too little information. Such surveys should have films of hands, feet, cervical spine, and — desirably — one knee. The readings should focus on joint groups rather than individual joints.

The second kind of survey that is needed is of a much more intensive nature and presumably should be undertaken at only a limited number of research centers. In such surveys, the maximum number of joints should be X-rayed, and each joint should be read individually. The purpose of this is to study patterns of joint involvement. For example, it is important to learn the extent to which osteoarthrosis of spinal interfacetal joints is correlated with peripheral osteoarthrosis as opposed to disk degeneration.

Third, a longitudinal study of a modest group should be undertaken to learn something of the natural evolution of osteoarthrosis. In addition to these field studies, there should be more epidemiology at the autopsy table. The loss from the biased samples obtained at autopsy is balanced by the gain of more detailed information on individual joints. Finally, it is clear that the last word has not been said on the causes of pain and swelling in osteoarthrosic joints.

It seems likely that epidemiology will continue to contribute to our knowledge of osteoarthrosis and disk degeneration. As our understanding of these conditions improves, it will become appropriate for us to evaluate the disability caused by them and the medical care required to manage them.

6 / GOUT AND HYPERURICEMIA

6.0 Introduction. The Disease. Gout is a metabolic disease the most striking manifestation of which is an excruciatingly painful form of arthritis. This comes in acute attacks, lasting a week or two, and may go on to a chronic deforming disease of the joints. It is sometimes associated with renal disease that can be fatal. The immediate mechanism of acute arthritis appears to be precipitation of uric acid crystals in the joint space and periarticular tissues. In the chronic form, the damage is done by the deposition of uric acid in tophi that destroy adjacent tissue as they grow.

Criteria for the diagnosis of gout in survey work were recommended by the Third International Symposium on Population Studies in the Rheumatic Diseases (Bennett and Burch, 1967):

The diagnosis of gout should be based upon: #1 or #2 below:
1. The demonstration of urate crystals in synovial fluid or of urate deposition in tissues by chemical or microscopical examination. The demonstration of uratic urinary calculi does not satisfy this criterion.
2. The presence of two or more of the following four criteria:
    a) A clear history (and/or observation) of attacks of painful, limb joint swelling. These attacks, at least in the early stages, must exhibit an abrupt onset of severe pain and complete clinical remission within a week or two.
    b) A clear history (and/or observation) of podagra, that is, an attack as described above involving the great toe.
    c) The presence of tophi.
    d) A clear history (and/or observation) of a good response to colchicine defined as a major reduction in objective signs of inflammation within 48 hours of the onset of therapy.
It is assumed that serum uric acid determinations will be carried out on the population under study, that a frequency distribution curve of the levels will be prepared, and that the levels of individuals found to meet any one or more of the criteria will be available.

The subcommittee does not propose that paracentesis (1) of all joints containing fluid be carried out in future survey work on gout. It also recognizes that the response on the effectiveness of colchicine (2nd) will vary rather more with the level of medical sophistication in a community than with the prevalence of gout. But if either type of information can be obtained, it should be recorded because of its high degree of specificity.

All survey work pertinent to gout should include responses to 2a, b, and c, on every individual examined.

These criteria represent a real advance because they permit an examination of the relation of urate level to clinical gout. They make no distinction between primary and secondary gout, largely because it is believed that secondary gout is only a small portion of total gout and is not practically separated out in field surveys.

Gout is a disease known in antiquity. In the fifth century B.C., Hieron of Syracuse commented on the association of joint disease and bladder stones. However, the earliest written account of gout is usually attributed to Hippocrates, who entitled it "the unwalkable disease." He wrote that it was incurable, that it appeared in the spring and fall, and that eunuchs were free of it, as were all women until after the menopause. In the second century A.D., Galen added that it was inheritable and related to luxurious eating and drinking. In 1783 Sydenham observed that those suffering from gout "generally have large heads, are of a full, humid, and lax habit, and possess a luxurious and vigorous constitution with excellent vital stamina." The history of gout and of the distinguished persons who have suffered from it is well presented in a variety of sources to which the interested reader is commended (Schnitker, 1936; Hormell, 1940; Hartung, 1957; Talbott, 1964).

6.1 Prevalence. The most useful measure of the frequency of gout is the prevalence of persons who have had one or more attacks of the disease referred to, for convenience, as the prevalence of gouty persons. There are two ways of estimating this parameter. Each has its advantages and disadvantages. The first is the population survey.

There are fifteen populations listed in Table 6.1, on which adequate information about the prevalence of gouty persons has been obtained. A cursory glance at this table reveals considerable variation in the estimated frequencies. It is suspected that much of the variation results from differences in method, differences in age distribution, and small sample sizes. The one thing that stands out is that the disease appears to be substantially and consistently more frequent among the Maoris of New Zealand than among other populations. On the basis of a hospital out-patient group, Fisher (1959) believes that gout is also excessively frequent among Filipinos. The next highest estimates are from the Polynesian Islands and Framingham, Massachusetts. This last survey covers a ten-year period, and thus is not really comparable to any of the others, in which the diagnoses were established at the time of a single examination. Although these comparisons are fraught with all sorts of methodologic problems, it seems likely that the frequency of gout is truly high in Maori and Polynesian populations because as will be seen below (section 6.5) the mean serum uric acid levels are also elevated in these groups.

Table 6.1   Prevalence of gouty persons by sex in various populations

Country and Study	Number of Persons Examined		Prevalence per 1,000	
	M	F	M	F
United States				
New York, N. Y., employees, 18–64 (Brown and Lingg, 1961)	5000	500	4.	–
Framingham, Mass., population, 40+ (Hall et al., 1967)	2283	2284	28.	4.
Tecumseh, Mich., population, 40+ (Dodge, 1964)	1557	1580	8.	5.
Blackfoot Indians, population, 30+ (Bennett and Burch, 1968e)	587	435	–	–
Pima Indians, population, 30+ (Bennett and Burch, 1968e)	473	475	4.	–
Great Britain				
Leigh, Lancs., population, 55–64 (Popert and Hewitt, 1962)	173	207	17.	–
Wensleydale, Yorkshire, population, 15+ (Popert and Hewitt, 1962)	485	540	–	–
Edinburgh, Scotland, dockyard, 15–64 (Anderson and Duthie, 1963)	1422	---	1.	---
New Zealand				
Maoris, Whanau-a-apanui, population "adults" (Lennane et al., 1960)	219	243	82.	16.
Maoris, Arawa, population, "adults" (Lennane et al., 1960)	83	103	60.	–
Non-Maori, Rotorua, population, "adults" (Lennane et al., 1960)	296	345	7.	–
Europeans, Carterton, population, 15+ (Rose et al., 1968)	202	228	20.	
Polynesia				
Rarotonga, population, 15+ (Rose et al., 1968)	243	227	24.	–
Pukapuka, population, 15+ (Rose et al., 1968)	188	191	53.	–
Japan				
Osaka, population, --- (Shichikawa and Komatsubara, 1964)	2500	2519	1.	–

Another way of estimating the prevalence of gouty persons is by looking for the disease in routine autopsy series. Such series are of course overbalanced with persons who are elderly, who die in hospitals, who have unusual diseases, and who die under suspicious circumstances. Nevertheless they do give another source from which to make reasonable estimates. Autopsy series in which joint disease has been systematically studied are relatively few. No attempt will be made to consider every one of these studies, but two series from Germany deserve mention.

Beitzke in 1912 and Heine in 1926, respectively, estimated the prevalence of gouty persons to be 40 and 11 per 1,000 persons autopsied. These estimates may be high, because special efforts may have been made to obtain permission for autopsy on persons with joint disease. Moreover, the prevalence of persons suffering from secondary gout is likely to be higher in such autopsy series than in the general population. On the other hand, estimates based on autopsy series are probably low, because not all cases of gout can be identified by autopsy, for only the chronic tophaceous form is recognizable pathologically.

To supplement these estimates, we have only a few clinical observations. Decker and Lane (1959) noted the frequency with which Filipinos came to the King County Hospital in Seattle with gout. Ford and deMos (1964) believe that gout, like hyperuricemia, is unduly frequent in the Chinese of British Columbia. Finally we have the strong clinical impressions of Das Gupta (1935) that the disease is very common in Nepal. This is confirmed by correspondence with E. R. Miller of the United Mission Hospital in Khatmandu, who emphasizes that "among the high class which constitutes about 5 percent of the population gout is quite frequent while among the 95 percent, the poorer class, gout is very infrequent."

Beyond this I can only say that we know of no race, no culture, and no portion of the earth that is entirely free of gout. There are many clinical reports, hospital reports, and informed impressions in the literature but these are no substitute for epidemiologic evidence. However, it is worth mentioning that fluctuations in the frequency of gout over time are a common subject for discussion among rheumatologists. The only documentation that I know of is from Tokyo (Oshima *et al.*, 1964). There is an evident need for more adequate prevalence estimates for this disease so that we can make comparisons between populations and through time.

6.2 Incidence. It has been estimated that the annual incidence of gout in Framingham and Sudbury, Massachusetts, is 0.1 percent (Hall *et al.*, 1964; O'Sullivan, 1968).

6.3 Associations. From the clinical literature it is quite clear that gout is more frequent in the male than in the female, and that females are rarely affected before the menopause. It is also clear that gout increases in frequency with age. Although clinical reports suggest that no races and no locations are entirely free of the disease, there appear to be secular trends in its frequency. And finally, there are strong persistent impressions that gout is more common in the upper than in the lower social classes. None of these points is adequately documented from an epidemiologic standpoint except for the sex difference, which was demonstrated in Table 6.1, and some data on age provided by Hall and his team in 1967. Since our present purpose is epidemiologic and statistical, no effort will be made to review the vast clinical literature that has accumulated from the time of Hippocrates to the present.

Clearly more adequate epidemiologic data is needed on the distribution of this disease by age, sex, race, place of residence, and social class.

6.4 Relation of Serum Uric Acid Level to Frequency of Gout. Since about 1800 it has been suspected that high levels of uric acid in the blood and urine are associated with gout (Talbott, 1964). In 1848 Garrod developed the thread test for hyperuricemia. In 1913 Folin and Dennis proposed the phosphotungstic colorimetric method, and by 1939 a highly specific method was available in the ultraviolet spectrophotometric uricase method (Blauch and Koch, 1939; Praetorius, 1949). The final step in this sequence was the suggestion that uric acid can be quantitated with considerable validity and reproducibility by an automated process (Bywaters and Holloway, 1964). However, O'Sullivan (1968) has pointed out that interlaboratory variation may still be appreciable.

Not until adequate biochemical methods were combined with large-scale population surveys could the hypothesis that the frequency of gout is a function of the level of uric acid in the serum be tested. At the present time we have two tests of this hypothesis. These are presented together in Table 6.2, which shows the prevalence of persons who have had one or more attacks that can be clearly called gout. The data are drawn from the Framingham Heart Study (Hall *et al.*, 1967) and from the Tecumseh Health Study (Dodge, 1964).

This table demonstrates several things. First, for each sex and for each study there is a systematic increase in the frequency of gout with increase in the level of urate in the serum. Second, the difference between the studies is more striking than the difference between the

Table 6.2　Prevalence of persons with gout by serum uric acid level at age 40 and over, by sex, in Framingham, Massachusetts, and Tecumseh, Michigan

Location, population, cases and rate	Serum uric acid level							
	Less than 6		6.0-6.9		7.0-7.9		8.0+	
	M	F	M	F	M	F	M	F
Framingham, Mass. exam. #2								
Population	1615	2405	354	71	78	11	22	1
Gout cases	18	3	26	5	11	3	8	-
Rate per 1,000	11	1	73	70	141	273	364	-
Tecumseh, Mich. exam. #1								
Population	712	876	177	69	56	33	31	12
Gout cases	3	2	-	2	4	2	4	-
Rate per 1,000	4	2	-	29	71	61	130	-
Overall rate per 1,000	5		49		112		182	

Source: Hall et al., 1967; Dodge, 1964.

sexes. This is probably methodologic in origin. Third, if one groups all the data for the two sexes and the two studies as in the last row, the relationship appears to be approximately linear.

Hall and his colleagues (1967) have also looked at the likelihood of gout and of renal lithiasis by maximum serum urate level during the entire period of observation of the Framingham study. An abstract of their data is presented in Table 6.3. While the data are incomplete for renal stones at the lower levels of serum uric acid and while the extent of overlap between gout and urolithiasis is not available, there is again the clear impression of a very great increase in both conditions as urate level advances. From a preventive-medicine standpoint this table has real importance, but the purpose here of presenting the table has been to lay out a fundamental principle in the investigation of gout.

Specifically, to really understand the epidemiology of gout those factors that elevate the serum uric acid must be separated from those factors that change the probability of an attack of gout at a given uric acid level. The best way to identify factors other than uric acid level that contribute to gout is to examine the shape of the curves of gout frequency against uric acid level for groups with and without the factors under consideration.

Table 6.3   The probability of having gout or renal lithi-
             asis before age 54 by the maximum of six serum
             uric acid determinations in the last 10 years,
             Framingham, Mass.

Maximum serum uric acid level in mg/ml	Number of persons	Percent with gout	Percent with renal stones
Under 6.0	3,946	0.3	-
6.0-6.9	941	2.	-
7.0-7.9	185	17.	9.
8.0-8.9	44	23.	18.
9.0 & over	11	82.	36.

Source: Hall et al., 1967.

Note: The sexes have been combined because the risk
is not related to sex except as uric acid levels differ in
the two sexes.

Rose and his fellow-workers (1968) have presented some data that
suggest that those Maoris living in Rarotonga are less likely to have
gout at 8 mg percent or over than are other Maoris living either in
Pukapuka or in New Zealand. The difference is both striking and
statistically significant, but the full data have never been presented in
a way to permit comparison with Table 6.2. There are two difficulties.
First, an appreciable number of New Zealand Maoris are on long-term
uricosuric medication and the handling of them in the tables is not
clear. Second, the authors have not, so far as I can determine, presented the full set of data on the frequency of gout by serum uric
acid class. Ideally, the data should be presented in such a way as to
permit plotting of the frequency of gout against uric acid level.

6.5 Serum Uric Acid Levels. Since there is a clear association of
high uric acid levels with the frequency of gout, serum surveys have
been made with some frequency. A variety of methods are available
for the determination of uric acid. Of these the ultraviolet spectrophotometric uricase method (Praetoris and Poulsen, 1953; Liddle
et al., 1959) is the most valid and reproducible. Unfortunately, it is

cumbersome and not easily adapted to mass-production methods; nevertheless it has been recommended as the standard for survey work (Brøchner-Mortensen *et al.*, 1963).

At the present time there are available reports on eight populations of substantial size in which this method has been used. The mean values for males and females are summarized in Table 6.4. The standard deviations for these groups and subgroups are consistently between 1.0 and 1.2 mg percent. These are all Caucasian populations, and as can be seen there is an extraordinary uniformity. Alper and Seitchik (1957) and Ford and deMos (1964) have used other methods but have properly calibrated them against the standard method, so that a correction factor is available. One wishes that all investigators would thus calibrate their methods. Ford's results on a grab sample of Canadians approximate the results in the table, but those of Alper give slightly higher results for a population of blood donors.

Most of the above data were collected around or before 1960. More recent studies in the United States seem to be producing higher levels. This is most strikingly true of the studies in New

Table 6.4   Mean serum uric acid levels as determined by the spectrophotometric uricase method for certain Caucasian populations

Population	Males, post-adolescent		Females	
	Cases	Mean SUA	Cases	Mean SUA
High school students, U.S. (Cobb, 1963)	138	5.2	74	4.0 [a]
Small community, U.S. (Mikkelsen et al., 1965)	573	5.2	720	4.0 [a]
Military recruits, U.S. (Stetten and Hearon, 1959)	817	5.1	-	-
"Normals," Denmark (Hauge and Harvald, 1955)	130	5.1	-	-
Hospital staff, Denmark (Gjørup et al., 1955)	143	5.0	157	3.8
Penitentiary, U.S. (Decker et al., 1962)	88	5.0	-	-
Rural community, England (Popert and Hewitt, 1962)	436	4.5	320	3.5 [a]
Urban community, England (Acheson and Lawrence, 1969)	158	5.0	163	4.4

[a] Female populations known to contain no persons over 45.

Haven, Connecticut (Acheson and O'Brien, 1966a) and Sudbury, Massachusetts (O'Sullivan, 1968). According to Duff *et al.* (1968), by the second round in Tecumseh, Michigan, the mean level had risen from the values given by Mikkelsen (1965) and shown in the table to 5.8 mg percent for men and 4.8 mg percent for women. A similar trend in successive studies in my own laboratory is apparent (Kasl *et al.*, 1968). I have looked at the literature and at continuous records from some hospitals and have found suggestive evidence of a secular trend to increasing levels over the last forty to fifty years, but the changes in method have made it almost impossible to be sure if this is really happening. Perhaps such a trend can now be documented or disproved. This will require interlaboratory standardization over a wide range of values or a return to the more cumbersome spectro-photometric uricase method.

High mean levels for serum urate have been found in Maoris (Lennane *et al.*, 1960), certain Polynesians (Burch *et al.*, 1966; Prior *et al.*, 1966), rural Malaysians (Duff *et al.*, 1968), and in Filipinos in the United States (Decker and Lane, 1959; Steuermann and Farias, 1960) but not in Filipinos remaining at home (Healey *et al.*, 1966). Similarly, Ford and deMos (1964) have found elevated levels in Chinese living in this country, but Duff and his associates (1968) suggest that Chinese from Taiwan and Malaya do not have levels appreciably above those current for Tecumseh, Michigan. Dreyfuss and his colleagues have compared levels among a variety of groups in the Middle East (1960, 1961, 1964).

By contrast, Jamaicans (Brenner and Lawrence, 1966) and American Indians of three different tribes (Ford and deMos, 1964; O'Brien *et al.*, 1966) do not differ appreciably from the Caucasian population analyzed in Table 6.3. Furthermore, it seems likely that the Japanese are not significantly different, although the data have been obtained by the colorimetric method (Shichikawa and Komatsubara, 1964).

At this point we should point out that there is far too much talk about the concept of hyperuricemia. The term is meaningless, because when it is used it is seldom made clear whether one is talking about some cutoff point in the upper ranges of the frequency distribution of the population in question, or whether one is talking about the solubility of uric acid in body fluids or about the likelihood of developing gout and urolithiasis. As we have seen in section 6.3, it makes little sense to set different levels for hyperuricemia for the two sexes if these levels are to be related to the diagnosis of gout, because the likelihood of gout seems clearly related to uric acid level and quite independent of sex when uric acid level is held constant. I would suggest that the concept of hyperuricemia be abandoned in favor of the more complex probability of disease statements in Tables 6.2 and 6.3. Specifically the data from Framingham, Massachusetts, presented in Table 6.3 suggest that a man whose serum uric acid level exceeds 9.0 milligrams percent has a probability of about 0.8 of having had an attack of gout and a probability of about 0.4 of having had a renal stone by the time he gets into his mid-fifties. The number of persons on which this estimate is based is small, but the implied risk is so high as to warrant serious attention.

6.6 Factors Associated with Uric Acid Level. There are a number of host factors that appear to influence the serum urate level. Prominent among these are age and sex. The best data on this matter come from the Tecumseh Community Health Study (Mikkelsen *et al.*, 1965) and are plotted in Figure 6.1. In both sexes the levels rise during adolescence. For boys the rate of the rise is quite steep, reaching

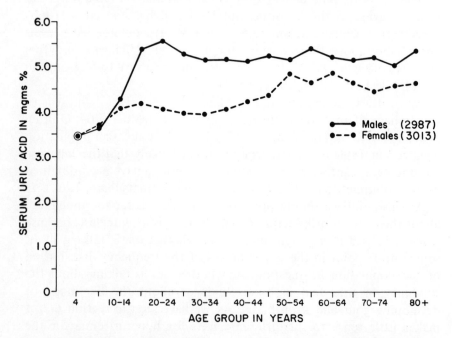

Fig. 6.1 Serum uric acid levels by age and sex. Tecumseh, Michigan, 1959 to 1960. (Reproduced with permission from Mikkelsen *et al.*, 1965.)

about 5 milligrams per milliliter in the early twenties at which level it persists for the rest of life. For girls the adolescent rise is more gradual, leveling out in the teens at approximately 4 milligrams per milliliter. At the time of the menopause the level rises again to approximate the level of the adult man. This obviously makes sense of the report by Hippocrates that women are not affected by gout until after the menopause.

Body weight and correlated measures of body size usually have been found to be associated with serum urate level (Burch *et al.,* 1966; O'Brien *et al.,* 1966; Acheson and O'Brien, 1966*a*; Healey *et al.,* 1966; Prior *et al.,* 1966; Bennett and Burch, 1968*e*). However, the association has not always been found and never accounts for a large amount of the variance (Cobb *et al.,* 1966*a*) although the slope of the regression line is great enough to be meaningful (Acheson and O'Brien, 1966*b*). One of the more noteworthy bits of data on this subject is presented in Table 6.5, which shows a rather striking increase in uric acid level with obesity.

For a long time it has been recognized clinically that polycythemia is related to elevated uric acid levels. Now Acheson and O'Brien (1966*a*) have shown that uric acid and hemoglobin levels are associated in the normal range. By the same token, leukemia has been recognized as involving high uric acid levels and another disease involving high turnover of white cells, infectious mononucleosis, also has

Table 6.5   Relationship between serum uric acid level and ratio of body weight to ideal weight at age 25 for 134 blue collar employees at a metal refining plant

Weight ratio	Number of cases	Mean uric acid level in mg/ml
0.90-0.99	15	4.2
1.00-1.19	68	4.8
1.20-1.29	33	5.1
1.30 +	18	5.7

Source: Mott et al., personal communication.

been shown to have elevated serum levels (Cowdrey, 1966). With the added information that vigorous exercise (Nichols *et al.,* 1951; Zachau-Christiansen, 1959) and starvation (Scott *et al.,* 1964; Shapiro *et al.,* 1964) also raise serum urate levels, one is led to the belief that perhaps we are dealing with the number of body cells destroyed per day.

In fact, the relation to body weight might also be accounted for in this way; for the larger the body, the greater the number of cells destroyed per day, the greater the amount of nucleic acid released, and thus the greater the amount of uric acid entering the system. One has to remember in formulating an hypothesis of this sort that it assumes a constant rate of elimination from the body, which is probably not the case (Yu *et al.,* 1957; Murphy and Shipman, 1963). We conclude that if we are to understand these matters fully it is important to measure urinary excretion rates as well as serum levels. Timed urine specimens are not impossible to obtain in field studies (Cobb *et al.,* 1966b); and in this connection it is well to remember that there are diurnal variations in the rate of urate excretion (Argen and Dixon, 1965).

On the matter of diet, it is a clinical fact that the serum urate of gout patients can be appreciably reduced by a low purine diet. Convincing evidence that the same is true for the normal individual has not been readily available. Dr. W. E. Reynolds (1969) says that he has performed experiments on normal persons in which he has produced substantial changes by drastic dietary measures; however, it does not seem likely that the usual interindividual variations in diet, among Caucasian people, account for much of the observed variation in level. Beyond this there are a wide variety of metabolities, especially ketones (Lecocq and McPharl, 1964) and drugs (Demartini, 1965), that influence urate levels and/or contribute to errors of measurement in uric acid assay. This is basically a clinical matter, but the list of potential hazards is long and the epidemiologist must beware.

The association of gout with high status occurs so regularly in history and in jest, as well as in the medical literature, that there is no need to document it. Still, it was only recently that research demonstrated that the mean serum uric acid level is higher for executives than it is for craftsmen (Dunn *et al.,* 1963). In this work serum urate level appears to be more related to the achieved social status of the individual than to that of his ancestors. Certainly social class by itself has not been consistently associated with uric acid level (Acheson and Lawrence, 1969).

In subsequent research, Brooks and Mueller (1966) have found that among university professors there is a correlation of 0.66 between a measure of drive, achievement, and leadership and the serum uric acid level. This seems to support the hypothesis of Orowan (1955) that uric acid, like its chemical relatives caffeine and theobromine, may be a cerebral stimulant. On the other hand, more recent work suggests that alternatively, or perhaps in addition, uric acid levels are influenced by stressful changes in the environment (Rahe and Arthur, 1967 and 1968; Kasl *et al.*, 1968). Studies aimed at further unraveling this relationship are much needed.

For the moment the most attractive hypothesis seems to me to be the notion that uric acid and/or its precursors xanthine and hypoxanthine are stimulants and that those people who respond well to environmental pressures are those whose uric acids go up in anticipation. If this hypothesis is correct, it is possible that the consumption of alcoholic beverages, which appears to be more frequent among those with high uric acids (Dawber *et al.*, 1964; Dodge and Mikkelson, 1964), may result at least in part from a desire for the sedative action of the alcohol. It must also be remembered that the consumption of alcohol has an indirect effect on the kidney via the blood-lactate level, which may cause retention of uric acid (Lieber, 1965).

Moore and Weiss (1963), after a review of the clinical literature, suggest that patients who have had a myocardial infarction have higher uric acid levels than persons who have not. I feel it is possible that the elevation of the uric acid level may follow the infarction, for uric acid levels were not found to be significant predictors of infarction in either the Framingham or Tecumseh studies (Dawber *et al.*, 1964; Dodge and Mikkelsen, 1964). Mikkelsen (1965) has been unable to substantiate his suspicion of an association between diabetes and gout in a population sample, although this relationship appears in a good many clinic samples.

6.7 Factors Precipitating Acute Gout. The immediate mechanism setting off the acute pain of gouty arthritis seems to be the sudden appearance of uric acid crystals in the joint space or periarticular tissues (Faires and McCarty, 1962; Seegmiller *et al.*, 1962). However, very little is known definitively about the nature of the events that can precipitate these crystals. Clearly the frequency of attacks increases with age. Attacks seem to occur at times of rapid change, either up or down, in serum urate levels (Maclachlan and Rodnan, 1967). Trauma, exposure, emotional arousal, allergy, lead poisoning, and overindulgence in food, alcohol, and sex have all been discussed at length by various clinical authors. There is great need for a longitudinal study of persons with high serum urate levels, to examine these matters in further detail.

6.8 Genetics. It has been a common observation from the beginnings of medicine to the present that gout appears to be hereditary; still, adequate evidence has been gathered only rather recently. It takes several forms. The first bit of evidence is that cited above, to the effect that there are certain races that appear to be unduly affected. The second is the long series of reports, beginning with the one by A. B. Garrod in 1848 and including at least a dozen in the English-language literature, which indicate that approximately 50 percent of persons with gout have a family history of the disease. Almost without exception these reports give no indication of a family history of gout among patients with other diseases or among well persons; the constant implication is that the frequency for gouty persons is higher than the authors would expect for nongouty persons.

The third type of evidence is derived from investigation of the relatives of persons with gout. The data of this type that I have been able to find are summarized in Table 6.6. On the top line, "Total of studies," a prevalence estimate across all studies is presented. The prevalence for individual studies is not calculated because the numbers are so small that very unreliable estimates would result. The

Table 6.6   Prevalence of persons with gout among the relatives of persons with gout

Studies	Number of relatives		Number with gout	
	M	F	M	F
Total of studies	474	425	62	11
Prevalence per 1,000			131	26
(Stecher, Hersh and Solomon, 1949)	25	31	3	0
(Hauge and Harvald, 1955)	130	131	15	1
(Popert and Hewitt, 1962)	2	4	2	0
(Rakic et al., 1964)	131	111	13	6
(Talbott, 1964) (review of 1940 study)	79	57	3	0
(Talbott, 1964) (case reports)	9	---	2	---
(Emmerson, 1960)	14	10	5	1
(Duncan and Dixon, 1960)	4	4	0	0
(Wilson, 1951)	30	25	13	3
(Bremner and Lawrence, 1966)	50	52	6	0

reports of Talbott (1940) and of Smyth and his associates (1948) have not been included because of the heavy overlap with later reports on the same kinships. Comparison of this table with Table 6.1 indicates immediately that persons with gout are substantially more common among the relatives of persons with gout than they are in the general population. The materials for Table 6.6 are not very satisfactory. In the future reports of such studies should be presented by degree of relatedness and by age.

The fourth kind of evidence is the demonstration that relatives of persons with gout tend to have higher mean serum uric acid levels than others. The simple reports of hyperuricemia in relatives are adequately summarized by Smyth (1957) and Kellgren (1964). More impressive evidence is found in the work of Neel and his team (1965), wherein it is demonstrated that the mean uric acid level is roughly dependent on the degree of relatedness to a person with gout; and in the work of Jensen *et al.* (1965) and Boyle *et al.* (1967), who found evidence for both hereditary and environmental influences in their twin studies. The logical final step has been taken by O'Brien and his co-workers (1966), with their calculation that the degree of heritability of uric acid levels in parent-child pairs of American Indians is approximately 20 percent. Similar estimates for Tecumseh, Michigan, by French *et al.* (1967) give a heritability of about 30 percent.

There has been much discussion of the mechanism by which the uric acid level is transmitted in families. Present opinion favors a polygenic influence (Neel *et al.,* 1965; O'Brien *et al.,* 1966). It should be noted, however, that the possibility of the influence of early life environment has not been adequately investigated, and a study in circumstances of communal child-rearing would be worthwhile.

6.9 Control Measures. It was pointed out in Tables 6.2 and 6.3 that there is a great excess of gout and urolithiasis in persons with serum uric acid levels of 8 mg percent or over. At 9 mg percent the risk becomes almost a certainty of developing one or the other disease, or both. Since both are very painful and disabling, it seems appropriate to consider routine screening procedures (Cobb, 1965*b*).

In the past, reliable uric acid determinations have been difficult to obtain, but a reasonably satisfactory automated process is now available (Bywaters and Holloway, 1964). This means that there is not only evidence of the value of screening for gout but the technical competence to do it. It is time that uric acid levels be included as routine for hospital admissions, periodic examinations, and multiple screening surveys, along with chest X-rays and tests for diabetes. This is particularly true for executives and university professors who are unduly prone to gout. Of course, persons with a family history of gout should have uric acids done from time to time.

When persons with elevated levels are detected there are two immediate considerations. First, has this person had an attack of gout or stone in the past, and what is his risk of having an attack in the future? For those with levels consistently above 8 mg percent, I believe that it is reasonable to consider the exhibition of uricosuric drugs because the risk of gout and renal stone is so high. As is seen in Table 6.3, of those with only their highest of six values between 8.0 and 8.9 mg. per ml., 23 percent have had an attack of gout and 18 percent have had a kidney stone by age 54. These are obviously overlapping risks for some persons suffer from both gout and stone. At 9.0 mg. per ml. and higher the percentages are so high as to suggest that to escape both gout and stone would be unusual. Combining the data to get an estimate of the risks among all those over 8.0 mg. per ml., we get 35 percent for gout and 22 percent for stone, and this is only for those intermittently over 8.0 mg. per ml. Presumably the estimated risks would be higher if they were based on levels consistently above 8.0 mg. per ml. and on longer periods of observation.

It is important that these estimates of risk be checked in other studies because if they are confirmed, physicians will have as much responsibility to prevent first as later attacks. Though it will probably never be practicable to prevent all acute attacks of gout, new cases of the chronic tophaceous form should not occur. This is largely the task of preventive medicine, but public health can assist by locating unrecognized cases.

6.10 Overview. Gout appears to be relatively rare in most populations; however, there are certain populations that have elevated uric acid levels and excessively frequent gout. It is clear that urate and gout are related and that they vary from population to population, but it is by no means clear that the relationship between these two variables is uniform across populations. More population studies are indicated. Uric acid levels are interestingly related to status, achievement, and environmental stress, but may in part be genetically determined. Finally, chronic tophaceous gout should occur rarely, if ever, in a society with adequate medical competence.

7 / THE CONNECTIVE-TISSUE DISORDERS

7.0 Introduction. This chapter will deal with polyarteritis nodosa, dermatomyositis, scleroderma, and lupus erythematosus. These are the more common of the connective-tissue disorders but they are much less common than those diseases that have come under scrutiny in previous chapters. Perhaps as a consequence of their rarity they have been less well studied, and certainly because of it they demand quite different epidemiologic approaches.

7.1 The Disorders. The most striking thing about the connective-tissue disorders is the extent to which they are interrelated with rheumatoid arthritis and with one another. The position is well stated by Copeman (1964):

It is often difficult or impossible to place a patient neatly in one or another diagnostic bracket: patients with many features of systemic lupus erythematosus may present features of scleroderma or dermatomyositis; polyarteritic changes may occur in all. The Hargraves (LE) cell phenomenon is seen typically in systemic lupus erythematosus, but is also seen in rheumatoid arthritis and occasionally in dermatomyositis or scleroderma. The sheep cell agglutination test, positive in most cases of rheumatoid arthritis, is also positive in many cases of systemic lupus erythematosus. So close may rheumatoid arthritis and systemic lupus erythematosus come together that some clinicians regard the latter as an extremely severe or malignant form of the former. Some workers consider that the vascular changes seen in rheumatoid arthritis, systemic lupus erythematosus, and polyarteritis nodosa can be distinguished from each other, but the spectrum of such changes is wide, and there is considerable overlap. . . The literature abounds in cases considered, on clinical or histological grounds, to be suffering at one point in time from one disorder and later on the same ground, from a different one.

In section 4.7 attention was called to the possibility that if there is an hereditary factor in these diseases, it might well be a general predisposition to develop one of the group rather than the diagnosis-specific type of heredity that has been sought in most studies.

7.2 Mortality is our principal way of assessing the frequency of these diseases. It is a valid criterion because these diseases are generally considered to be fatal; that is, they each appear to carry a prognosis involving a very substantial reduction in life expectancy. Life-table studies have been reported for lupus erythematosus (Merrell and Shulman, 1955; Kellum and Haserick, 1964), and it is hoped that soon there will be series of sufficient size that such studies can be carried out on the other diseases.

While these diseases have a high case fatality rate, we must assume that there are many missed cases. In order to show the order of magnitude of the mortality rates by age and sex, Table 7.1 has been prepared for the United States for the years 1959 to 1961. It required special coding by the National Center for Health Statistics and is probably the first time that national mortality data have been available for these diseases separately. Rheumatoid arthritis is included for comparison and in recognition of the fact that at autopsy some cases of rheumatoid arthritis may resemble other diseases in this group, especially polyarteritis (Ball, 1968).

The first thing that catches the eye in this table is that polyarteritis nodosa is consistently more common as a cause of death in men, whereas the other diseases cause more deaths in women. Second, it is notable that while rheumatoid arthritis appears as a cause of death with increasing frequency right into the oldest age groups, the other diseases begin to fall off somewhat as the years advance. Third, the age distribution of mortality in systemic lupus erythematosus is quite different for males and females. While males have their maximum mortality from the disease at about age 65, females hit their peak mortality at about 40. This might prove to be an epidemiologic fact of some importance.

In Table 7.2 are presented adjusted mortality rates for the same set of diseases by sex and race, by marital status, and by region in the United States. The adjustments were carried out by calculating, then summing, the number of deaths to be expected in each of the relevant age, sex, race, and region cells if the rates for the entire country were to prevail. This expected number was then divided into the number observed, and the result multiplied by the rate for the whole United States. Confidence limits for such ratios can be estimated from the table in Appendix C of Haenszel *et al.* (1962). While mentioned in the text, they would take up so much space in this table as to detract from its readability. From this table a number of things are evident:

(a) The excess of polyarteritis nodosa deaths in males noted in Table 7.1 is not found in the nonwhite males. In fact, the 95 percent confidence intervals for white and nonwhite males do not overlap.

Table 7.1 Mortality rates by age and sex for selected rheumatic diseases: United States, 1959–1961

Age group	Person years (millions)[a]		Mortality Rate per Million Person Years									
			Polyarteritis nodosa		Dermatomyositis		Scleroderma		Lupus erythematosus		Rheumatoid arthritis	
	M	F	M	F	M	F	M	F	M	F	M	F
All ages	265	273	1.8	1.2	0.3	0.6	1.1	2.4	1.1	4.7	4.6	9.1
Under 15	85	82	0.1	0.0	0.1	0.2	0.0	0.1	0.2	0.6	0.1	0.2
15–24	36	36	0.4	0.3	0.1	0.5	0.1	0.4	1.0	6.4	0.1	0.3
25–34	34	35	1.0	0.6	0.2	0.2	0.3	1.4	0.8	6.8	0.6	0.7
35–44	35	37	2.3	1.2	0.2	0.7	1.4	3.5	1.3	8.0	1.4	1.8
45–54	30	31	3.9	2.1	0.4	1.1	2.6	5.4	2.4	7.0	5.8	7.0
55–64	23	24	5.9	3.9	0.9	1.6	3.3	6.1	2.4	5.6	13.9	21.0
65–74	15	18	5.2	3.4	1.0	1.3	3.9	5.7	2.4	4.7	26.0	48.7
75 & over	7	10	2.0	1.5	1.1	0.9	1.1	3.1	1.7	2.7	33.4	80.7

Source: National Center for Health Statistics.

a Population of April 1, 1960, multiplied by three.

Table 7.2 Adjusted mortality rates by sex and color, marital status, and geographic region for selected rheumatic diseases United States, 1959-1961

Color, sex, marital status, and region	Person years (millions)	Adjusted mortality rates per million person years[a]				
		Polyarteritis nodosa	Dermato-myositis	Sclero-derma	Lupus erythematosus	Rheumatoid arthritis
Total U.S.A.	535[b]	1.5	0.5	1.8	2.9	6.8
White males	234	1.9	0.3	1.0	1.1	5.0
White females	241	1.1	0.6	2.1	4.0	8.8
Nonwhite males	29	1.2	0.4	2.1	1.8	3.3
Nonwhite females	31	1.3	1.2	4.7	10.6	5.9
Married[c]	257	2.1	0.6	2.4	3.7	8.8
Widowed[c]	30	1.7	0.6	2.5	4.4	9.7
Divorced[c]	9	3.2	0.8	3.4	6.2	13.0
Never married[c]	75	2.6	1.2	2.9	6.0	15.8
New England States	32	1.5	0.6	1.6	2.6	5.3
Middle Atlantic States	103	1.5	0.4	1.9	2.7	5.4
East North Central States	109	1.5	0.5	1.6	3.3	6.9
West North Central States	46	1.6	0.4	1.7	2.9	6.3
South Atlantic States	78	1.6	0.5	2.0	2.4	8.5
East South Central States	36	1.4	0.3	1.5	2.7	8.9
West South Central States	51	1.1	0.4	1.7	2.7	7.1
Mountain States	21	1.7	0.6	2.1	4.8	12.1
Pacific States	61	1.6	0.7	1.8	3.4	6.5

Source: National Center for Health Statistics.

a Ratio of observed to expected deaths multiplied by total U.S. death rate for that disease. See text.

b Population of April 1, 1960, multiplied by three.

c Age 15 and over.

(b) For dermatomyositis, scleroderma, and systemic lupus erythematosus, the highest mortality rates are found in the nonwhite females.

(c) For every one of these diseases, the divorced and the never-married have higher rates than the married and widowed. This extraordinary regularity deserves some investigation, for the differences are rather too large to result from any conceivable census error in classification by marital state, although Berkson (1962) has suggested such a possibility.

(d) The people of the Mountain states die with unusual frequency from these diseases. Specifically, for all of the diseases except dermatomyositis the rates are highest in the Mountain states (for dermatomyositis the numbers are small and the Mountain states rank second after the Pacific states). For rheumatoid arthritis and for systemic lupus erythematosus, the mean for all the other regions lies below the lower limits of the respective 95 percent confidence intervals for the Mountain states. The notion that this excess might be caused by people with these diseases migrating to Arizona and New Mexico was considered and found untenable because the rates in Montana and Idaho are about as high as the rates for the southern states in this region. The data were then examined for a tendency for mortality to occur at younger ages in the Mountain states. This tendency was striking only for systemic lupus erythematosus in women. Here the median age at death dropped from 40 for the United States as a whole to 33 for the Mountain states.

This suggestion of a geographic difference seems worthy of further study.

7.3 *Polyarteritis Nodosa* has received very little epidemiologic attention; however, a few quasi-epidemiologic studies are worthy of mention. In 1925 Gruber suggested on the basis of a careful review of the literature that this disease might be due to hypersensitivity. Ten years later Kline and Young (1935) presented three cases and said, "The picture suggests reactions to the same allergens as cause the usual clinical allergies." Then in 1942 Rich reported seven cases, five of which appeared to result from hypersensitivity to horse serum and two of which seemed to be related to sulfonamides. Since that time, there has been a long list of case reports suggesting hypersensitivity to various drugs, especially antibiotics. The association with antibiotic use again raises the question of the role of infection that was first brought up by Spiegel in 1936. This is clearly a field in which some good hospital-based epidemiology would be worthwhile. Also, the overlap of this disease with rheumatoid arthritis (Ball, 1968) deserves attention.

7.4 Dermatomyositis and Scleroderma are not only included in the same rubric in the International Statistical Classification of Disease, but appear to be interwoven in their manifestations (Medsger *et al.,* 1968) and were shown above to be reasonably similar in their mortality patterns. No further epidemiologic information about dermatomyositis has been uncovered, but scleroderma has received some attention. The age, sex, and race patterns of mortality for scleroderma noted in section 7.2 are very similar to those reported by Masi and D'Angelo (1967) for Baltimore, Maryland. The only other intriguing observation to date is that miners might be at some excess risk of the disease (Erasmus, 1957; Rodnan, 1963). Masi and D'Angelo (1967) looked for socioeconomic differences between their cases and controls but were unable to establish clear relationships. They suggest that the reporting of this disease on death certificates might be about 70 percent of the known cases. And who knows how many cases go undiagnosed?

7.5 Lupus Erythematosus. This disease is commonly referred to as systemic lupus erythematosus. I have, however, elected the terminology of Dubois (1966) in order to emphasize my agreement with his point that the discoid and the systemic forms of the disease are inseparable on any dimension other than prognosis and that much of what is called discoid today will be disseminated tomorrow.

Lupus erythematosus has had rather more epidemiologic study than the other diseases of this group, mostly as a result of the interest and vigor of Morris Siegel. First it should be noted that his figures (Siegel and Lee, 1968) for mortality from this disease in New York City are somewhat higher than the national figures given in Tables 7.1 and 7.2. This may simply be the result of better diagnosis in a sophisticated metropolitan area. By the same token, the discovery rates in Rochester, Minnesota, the home of the L.E. cell test, are substantially higher than the discovery rates in New York City (Nobrega *et al.,* 1968). Furthermore, increases in discovery rates over time have been noted in New York (Siegel and Lee, 1968) in Rochester, Minnesota (Nobrega *et al.,* 1968), and in Gothenburg, Sweden (Svanborg and Sölvell, 1957).

I use the term *discovery rate* here to emphasize that I do not believe these studies measure incidence, which is related to onset rather than diagnosis. My point is that epidemiology is just beginning with regard to this disease; we do not as yet have agreed-upon diagnostic criteria (Reynolds, 1968), and our ability to recognize the disease in its early and mild states is increasing by leaps and bounds. It is therefore important to be cautious in interpreting the available data. In any case, it is worthy of note that prevalence estimates for this disease reached 81 per million for New York City in 1964 (Siegel and Lee, 1968) and 418 per million in Rochester, Minnesota (Nobrega *et al.,* 1968), in 1966, and yet the disease appears not to have been identified in natives of Africa (Trowell, 1960).

With these cautions in mind, it is appropriate to call attention to certain bits of epidemiologic information. First, the morbidity data (Siegel and Lee, 1968) conform in pattern to the age, sex, and race distribution that appears in the mortality data presented in Tables 7.1 and 7.2. Specifically the disease is most prevalent in young and middle-aged nonwhite females. In addition, the data show an excess among Puerto Ricans as well as Negroes, but this does not appear to be simply a social-class phenomenon. Siegel and his associates (1967) have pointed out that drug-induced disease does not seem to have a predilection for the nonwhite, although it does seem to affect women more frequently than one would expect on the basis of the estimated frequency of administration of the drugs in question. The drugs most commonly involved are diphenylhydantoin, isoniazid, hydralazine, and procainamide.

As in rheumatoid arthritis, there may be an association with infectious processes. Dubois (1966) has called attention to what looks like an undue proportion of deaths from septicemia, pulmonary tuberculosis, and other infectious processes, and Myers and his fellow-workers (1967) have suggested that this increased susceptibility to infection may be more part of the disease than a result of steroid therapy. A further similarity to rheumatoid arthritis has been noted by Otto and Mackay (1967) in their work on the psychological and social factors that appear to contribute. Finally, Masi (1968) has reviewed the genetic literature on this disease and has come to no clear conclusion. The suggestion in Chapter 4 that perhaps we should be looking for a genetic factor increasing susceptibility to this disease and others of the collagen group applies here and is supported by the work of Siegel and his associates (1965), but not by that of Ansell and Lawrence (1963).

7.6 Overview. In this chapter we have noted the striking inter-relationships and similarities among these connective-tissue diseases and with rheumatoid arthritis. New data have been provided on the mortality from these diseases. We have looked at the rather scanty epidemiologic information on polyarteritis nodosa, dermatomyositis, and scleroderma, and have summarized the burgeoning epidemiology of lupus erythematosus. It is hoped that before long our clinical understanding of lupus erythematosus will stabilize enough to permit a committee to agree on diagnostic criteria to be used for epidemiologic purposes.

8 / ANKYLOSING SPONDYLITIS AND JUVENILE ARTHRITIS

8.0 Introduction. It is appropriate to deal with these conditions in the same chapter, for not only do they both have a relation to rheumatoid arthritis but also they have involvement of the sacroiliac joints in common (Bywaters and Ansell, 1965). Furthermore, there seems to be some familial association of the two diseases (Whittinghill *et al.,* 1958; Ansell *et al.,* 1968). We shall first discuss ankylosing spondylitis, then proceed to examine juvenile rheumatoid arthritis.

8.1 Ankylosing Spondylitis, according to Blumberg and Ragan (1956) is "an affliction primarily of young men, characterized by back pain and deformity resulting from involvement of the sacroiliac and small joints of the spine, paravertebral calcification and, in advanced cases, bony ankylosis of these regions." Diagnostic criteria for survey use have been proposed (Bennett and Burch, 1967) as follows:

Clinical criteria
1. Limitation of motion of the lumbar spine in all three planes — anterior flexion, lateral flexion, and extension.
2. A history of or the presence of pain at the dorso-lumbar junction or in the lumbar spine.
3. Limitation of chest expansion to 1 in. (2.5 cm.) or less, measured at the level of the fourth intercostal space.

Grading of radiographs
The sacroiliac joints on either side should be graded separately.
0 normal.
1 suspicious changes.
2 minimal abnormality — small localized areas with erosion or sclerosis, without alteration in the joint width.
3 unequivocal abnormality — moderate or advanced sacroiliitis with one or more of: erosions, evidence of sclerosis, widening, narrowing, or partial ankylosis.
4 total ankylosis.
For analysis the more severely affected joint should be considered, but a note should be made where the involvement is unilateral.

Application of these criteria
It is recommended that the frequency of occurrence of each criterion be reported separately, but for purposes of comparisons between surveys AS shall be defined by radiographic sacroiliitis accompanied by physical signs in the back.

Definite AS shall be present if there is grade 3-4 bilateral sacroiliitis with at least one clinical criterion, or if there is grade 3-4 unilateral or grade 2 bilateral sacroiliitis with clinical criterion 1 or with both clinical criteria 2 and 3.

Probable AS shall be present if there is grade 3-4 bilateral sacroiliitis without any clinical criteria.

When sacroiliitis is present, the following variants of AS should be designated individually: RA, psoriasis, ulcerative colitis or regional ileitis, Reiter's syndrome, and juvenile RA.

Individuals with conditions such as fluorosis, hypophosphatemic osteomalacia, brucellosis, and familial Mediterranean fever, which may confuse the picture of AS, should be identified in tabulations for AS and should be listed separately.

In the United States there is a tendency to refer to this disease as rheumatoid spondylitis, with the implication that it is related to rheumatoid disease. This is not the place to review all the arguments for and against the notion that these are two variants of the same disease, but it is worth reminding ourselves that epidemiologically they are quite distinct in their age, sex, and geographic distributions; this is true despite the fact that a disproportionate number of persons with obvious rheumatoid arthritis have sacroiliac involvement, and that persons with obvious ankylosing spondylitis have peripheral poly-arthritis with undue frequency.

8.2 Observer Variation in the reading of X-ray films of the sacro-iliac joints is considerable. The extent of this variation in one study involving competent physicians is presented in Table 8.1. The agreement on positives presumably can be improved with training of the

Table 8.1   Observer variation among three physicians reading X-rays of the sacroiliac joints for evidence of ankylosing spondylitis

Pair of observers	Agreement on positives for		
	Grade 4	Grade 3-4	Grade 2-4
A vs. B	8/21	15/40	37/64
A vs. C	9/21	16/43	35/67
B vs. C	7/10	12/24	30/62

Source: Gofton, 1966.

observers. At the moment, the level of agreement is not such as to inspire confidence in the reports of studies in which the sacroiliac films were read by a single observer. In future studies the X-ray readers should be carefully trained on other films before starting to read the films of the survey in question, and all films should be read more than once.

8.3 Prevalence. Until quite recently there have been no really useful estimates of the prevalence of ankylosing spondylitis. The information prior to 1956 is well reviewed by Blumberg and Ragan (1956), who properly conclude that it is difficult to determine the true frequency of the disease from the data available. By 1963 Kellgren (1964) was able to present data from six studies in the United States and Northern Europe indicating that for these populations the prevalence of clinical ankylosing spondylitis might well lie between 0.1 and 0.2 percent. Further, Mikkelsen and his colleagues (1967) report just over 0.2 percent for Tecumseh, Michigan.

Since that time the whole matter has been given a great deal of thoughtful study, and diagnostic criteria have been proposed for discussion and evaluation (Bennett and Burch, 1967). It has become clear that very specific comparisons need to be made if we are to detect geographic variations. With this in mind, Gofton and his co-workers (1966) have jointly read the pelvic X-rays from eight different male populations. The material is presented in admirable detail, and age-adjusted comparisons are made between the several Indian tribes. The overall comparisons are readily seen from Table 8.2 which is derived from their data, omitting only the data from the family study.

The calculation of rates from this table should be limited to the age group 55 and over, in which data are available on all the populations. The overall prevalence estimate for this group emerges as 3.8 percent. The data are really too thin to warrant age-adjusted comparisons, but the full detail is presented so that the reader can study the material for himself. From the last row it is evident that only two populations are clearly different from the rest. First, the Haida Indians have consistently higher rates than all the other populations. Of course, the Wensleydale figures seem a little high, but it is hard to know if they should be considered as indicating an important variation in the frequency within England. Despite the fact that the Wensleydale estimate is significantly higher than the Leigh figure (P<0.01), I tend to be cautious about interpretation. Of course, the

Table 8.2 The frequency of agreed upon sacroiliac (S-I) changes indicative of ankylosing spondylitis in seven male populations by age, changes of grade 2-4 according to the Atlas of Standard Radiographs based on A-P films of the pelvis read by three observers

Age, number of exams, & S-I changes		Haida Indians, USA	Wensley- dale, England	Pima Indians, USA	Watford, England	Blackfeet Indians, USA	Leigh, England	Jamaica, BWI
25-34								
	Exams	32	---	44	20	72	---	---
	S-I changes	1		-	-	1		
35-44								
	Exams	31	---	81	14	109	---	86
	S-I changes	3		2	-	4		-
45-54								
	Exams	34	---	68	28	93	---	83
	S-I changes	4		6	-	2		-
55-64								
	Exams	31	43	70	23	83	164	86
	S-I changes	3	4	2	1	3	3	-
65+								
	Exams	19	49	92	13	64	63	---
	S-I changes	3	2	4	-	1	1	
55+								
	Exams	50	92	162	36	147	227	---
	S-I changes	6	6	6	1	4	4	

Source: Gofton et al., 1966.

highest rate for sacroiliac changes suggesting ankylosing spondylitis is reported from ancient Egyptian remains (Ruffer, 1921).

Second, the Jamaica Negroes appear to have an appreciably lower rate than other populations, for no sacroiliitis was found among the 255 men X-rayed. This observation is particularly remarkable in view of the high rate of erosive arthritis of peripheral joints found in this population, and constitutes epidemiologic evidence that ankylosing spondylitis and rheumatoid arthritis are separate diseases.

Further studies of spondylitis should be undertaken among the Indians of the northwest coast of North America. There in that population the disease seems to be sufficiently frequent for some of the characteristics of its distribution to be revealed by a study of manageable size. Additional searches for geographic variation may prove profitable.

8.4 Association with Other Diseases. As with rheumatoid arthritis, we find that ankylosing spondylitis has important associations with other diseases. First Kellgren (1964) has reviewed seven studies in the period 1958 to 1964, each of which indicates an excess of clinical ankylosing spondylitis among persons with ulcerative colitis or regional ileitis. The frequency of spondylitis in these series ranges from 2.3 to 6.0 percent, or roughly ten to thirty times the usual frequency in Caucasian populations of similar age and sex distribution. Wright and Watkinson (1965) present further evidence supporting this association.

There is considerable clinical literature suggesting association with genito-urinary infection (Romanus, 1953), with prostatitis (Mason et al., (1958), and with anterior uveitis and genital infection (Caterall, 1960). These associations are strong enough so that they can hardly be a result of Berkson's (1946) fallacy. Romanus's point of view that the prostatitis cause the ankylosing spondylitis is not supported by a clearly sequential relationship between the two conditions. For the time being it is better to adhere to the limited conclusions of association. This is an appropriate matter for further study, perhaps in a military setting which would permit the identification of cases of genital infection and their follow-up in later life. The finding of sacroiliitis in patients with Reiter's disease is not really indicative of an association of the two diseases because the course is quite different (Good, 1965).

8.5 Heredity. The literature on this subject through 1963 is well covered by Kellgren in his Heberden Oration (1964). He points out that in the seven studies up to that time ankylosing spondylitis occurs about ten times as frequently among the relatives of cases as in the general population. Similar findings are reported by Emery and Lawrence (1967). These are larger differences than those found in similar studies of rheumatoid arthritis. The criticisms of this type of study that have been noted in the case of rheumatoid arthritis (Schull and Cobb, 1969) apply here, but the larger differences make it less likely that they account for the whole effect. Furthermore, two studies demonstrate the frequency of the disease by degree of consanguinity. Whittinghill et al. (1959) studied a kindred of some 3,300 people and nearly 1,800 controls, while de Blécourt and his associates (1961) studied about 2,500 relatives and some 2,400 controls. The data from these two studies are presented in Table 8.3, and are sufficiently striking to make one believe that inheritance accounts for a modest proportion of the variance in the distribution of this disease. It would of course be desirable to separate by sex, but such data are not available from Whittinghill and the data of de Blécourt become a little too thin when subdivided.

Table 8.3   The prevalence per 100 persons of ankylosing spondylitis among relatives of patients with that disease by degree of relatedness

Author	Degree of relatedness			
	First Degree	Second Degree	Third Degree	Unrelated
(Wittinghill, 1959)	6.3	2.9	0.7	0.1
(de Blécourt, 1961)	4.6	1.1	0.7	0.1

It is probably too early to know how to interpret the complex inheritance patterns suggested by the interrelationships with other diseases. For example, Whittinghill *et al.* (1959) suggests a genetic relationship between ankylosing spondylitis and juvenile rheumatoid arthritis but no genetic relationship of these two with rheumatoid arthritis, whereas Ansell and her fellow workers (1968) suggest that juvenile rheumatoid arthritis may be genetically associated with both peripheral and spinal arthritis. Perhaps the best interpretation is simply to take this as further evidence that we have not yet identified the relevant genetic marker or markers which predispose to a variety of rheumatic diseases.

8.6 Juvenile Rheumatoid Arthritis is presently thought to be simply the different expression of rheumatoid arthritis that is characteristic of the age group under 16 (Bywaters, 1967). The clinical differences between the juvenile and adult syndromes are well summarized by Calabro and Marchesano (1967). Despite the opinion of Ansell and Bywaters (1963) that no useful purpose is served by trying to subdivide the syndrome, the epidemiologist's eye cannot fail to be arrested by the observation of Calabro and Marchesano (1968) that there are age and sex differences between subgroups. The acute type with many systemic features has a sex ratio, M/F, of about 1.2 and mean age of onset of 4.6 years; the polyarticular type with a sex ratio of 0.6 has a mean age of onset of 7.4 years; and the monarticular type has a sex ratio of about 0.4 and a mean age of onset of 7.3 years. In a way the groupings look like severity groupings and we may be back to the observation of section 4.1, that the sex ratio for adult rheumatoid arthritis is about 1.0 for the severe cases while females predominate in the cases of moderate severity.

Bywaters (1968) has summarized the various attempts at devising diagnostic criteria for this disease, and his committee at the Third International Symposium has presented a proposed set for use in population surveys (Bennett and Burch, 1967). Because of the rarity of this disease it is difficult to imagine each person being examined in population surveys of the magnitude necessary to evaluate prevalence. Rather most surveys will have to be made using hospital records, school nurses, crippled-children's clinics, and the like as screening devices to identify the cases in a population. On the whole, multiple sources with collation to eliminate duplication will prove most satisfactory.

Before closing this section, it would be well to note that although the prognosis is on the whole good, Calabro and Marachesano (1968) an occasional patient dies, some go on to look much like adult rheumatoids, and a rare case, usually male, develops into classical spondylitis. Furthermore, some cases in which the diagnosis is only probable turn out to have lupus erythematosus or other rare but related diseases (Bywaters, 1967).

8.7 Onset. While the onsets in mild cases and those with insidious beginnings are hard to date, the distribution of onsets by sex is interesting and not likely to be biased except by the excess of the mild monarticular form in girls. Figure 8.1 shows the distribution of onsets found by Ansell and Bywaters (1963). The changing sex ratio with age has the same eye-catching properties as the changing ratio with severity. Since this sharp variation in sex ratio with age was not found by Sury (1952), more attention to this matter is indicated.

8.8 Mortality. The mortality attributed to rheumatoid arthritis in this age group is shown in Table 7.1 and is slightly in excess of one per ten million persons under age 15; it appears to be slightly greater for females than for males although the numbers are rather small to be sure of this. The principal cause of death in both Bywaters' (1967) and Barkin's (1952) series seems to be infection. However, heart disease was prominent in Barkin's (1952) and Sury's (1952) series, and infection did not appear in the latter's list of causes of death.

8.9 Prevalence and Incidence. Manheimer and his colleagues (1959) were able to identify 113 cases of rheumatoid arthritis under age 19 from hospital records in New York City. This yielded a point prevalence of 5 per 100,000. The authors made no claim to have identified

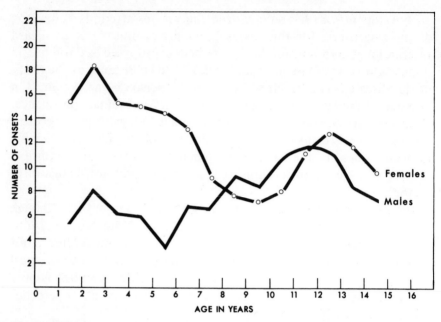

Fig. 8.1 Distribution of onsets among hospital cases of juvenile rheumatoid arthritis by age and sex, three-year moving averages calculated from Ansell and Bywaters (1963).

all the cases in this study that was designed for another purpose. Using data from hospitals and crippled children's clinics in Ohio, Gauchat (1957) estimated about 8 per 100,000. In England, Bywaters (1968) estimated 60 per 100,000 based on the referral of forty-three cases from a population of 66,000 school children in the districts adjoining Taplow. Den Ousten (1966) tells me that he found one case in 3,513 Dutch school children suggesting a prevalence estimate of about 30 per 100,000.

Finally, we have one estimate of annual incidence, perhaps more properly called annual discovery rate. It is for the city of Copenhagen by Sury (1952) and comes to 2.7 per 100,000 per year. Clearly, more incidence and prevalence data are required.

8.10 Heredity. Ansell and her colleagues are the only ones to have done a substantial analysis of the familial aspects of juvenile rheumatoid arthritis. The latest report from this study (Ansell *et al.,* 1968) suggests that the aggregation of sacroiliitis and peripheral arthritis occurred in the relatives of patients who had disease that remained active for five years or more, but was not found in the families of the milder cases. This resembles the finding noted above that rheumatoid arthritis aggregates, if at all, only in the families of the most severe cases. There was no aggregation of rheumatoid factor in these families.

The findings further support the importance of inclusive looks at all members of broad groups of connective-tissue diseases in the families of persons with one or another of these diseases. For this purpose I believe that rheumatic fever should be included with juvenile rheumatoid arthritis, spondylitis, rheumatoid arthritis, and the rarer connective-tissue diseases discussed in Chapter 7. This concept was used in the family study of Sjøgren's syndrome by Burch and his colleagues (1963) and should be more widely adopted. Nothing will be lost by this kind of approach and much may be gained.

8.11 Environmental Factors. The data in this area are uncontrolled clinical reports of the frequency with which infection and trauma have been noted in association with onset, plus some data on psychological and social factors. Unfortunately, final reports have never been published on the two best studies of psychosocial factors, and many of those who have studied the disease most carefully have neglected this area entirely. However, a few suggestions for further research have emerged.

In a clinical psychological study comparing the families of ten cases of juvenile rheumatoid arthritis with the families of ten cases of emotionally disturbed children and ten children doing well in the local grade school, it proved impossible to match on social class because the families of the juvenile rheumatoids were so low in comparison to the other two groups (Morris and Cobb, unpublished). From this study emerged only one very clear finding: going back to the time of conception of the case of juvenile rheumatoid disease and often back into the childhood of the parents, there simply was no pleasure to be found in the life of the patient or his family. This was in very sharp contrast to the other two groups and fits with the mentions of depression and resentment in the work of Blom and Whipple (1959), Grokoest *et al.* (1962), and Cleveland *et al.* (1965). Blom and Whipple go so far as to say, "Many of the mothers stated that the unhappiness or illness they had experienced during their pregnancy with the patient had affected the child and somehow had resulted in rheumatoid arthritis." It is my view that this is an opinion or rather an hypothesis that deserves attention.

In addition, Cleveland and his associates (1965) have demonstrated that children — like adults — with this disease have high barrier scores, presumably indicating a well-circumscribed and defended body image. They also have noted the tendency for these children to be active and "unusually expressive in physical and muscle action" up to the time their arthritis interferes. These are straws in the wind that deserve attention if we are to unravel the complex etiology of this disease.

8.12 Overview. Comparisons of the frequency of ankylosing spondylitis in various populations appear to be best made on the basis of X-rays of the sacroiliac joints, but such X-rays require duplicate readings because of the large observer variation involved. Substantial differences in frequency between populations have been noted, along with familial clustering of potential significance. With regard to juvenile rheumatoid arthritis, there are relatively few data. There is a rough estimate that the frequency of the disease is slightly less than 1 per 1,000 children; and there is some evidence that there may be a familial clustering with related diseases, and a pattern of relationships to the environment suggesting association with infection, injury, and pleasure deprivation.

9 / CODA

9.0 Introduction. In the several chapters that have gone before, detailed information has been provided about the frequency of each of the major rheumatic diseases. It now remains to view them in relation to one another and to the whole spectrum of disease. After that will come a final overview and a note on directions for the future.

9.1 Relative Disability and Need for Care. About 9 percent of the days lost from work in light industry result from arthritis and rheumatism (Brown and Lingg, 1961; Partridge *et al.,* 1965) and clearly more than this in mines and dockyards (Lawrence and Aitken-Swan, 1952; Anderson *et al.,* 1962; Anderson and Duthie, 1963). Similarly, as indicated in section 2.4, about 8 percent of the cases of illness, 4 percent of the doctors-office visits, and a little over 1 percent of the hospitalizations arise from rheumatic complaints.

It would be useful if we could distribute these by diagnosis. The only American information available other than the frequency distributions of diagnoses in arthritis clinics (for example, Lewis-Faning and Fletcher, 1945) comes from Brown and Lingg (1961). Their data suggest that in a working population of males, degenerative joint disease causes the most absences among the diagnosable complaints. However, they reported 54 percent of the absences as caused by other, undefined, or questionable rheumatic problems.

In a random sample of 1,342 persons from Leigh in northwest England, Lawrence (1965*b*) reports the distribution of days lost from school or work since birth, changes in job because of rheumatism, and total incapacity as shown in Table 9.1. Here it is evident that rheumatoid arthritis is the most important disabler among women, whereas disk disease leads the list for men.

Again from England, a detailed breakdown of days of sickness by age, sex, and arthritic diagnosis for 90,891 insured persons is available (Ministry of Health, 1924). The style of presentation is commendable and should be imitated. The data are not reproduced here because they are forty-five years old, and substantial progress in classification has been made in the interval.

Logan and Cushion (1958) did a year-long study of 106 general practices in England and Wales and provided useful data on consulta-

Table 9.1 Disability due to arthritis and rheumatism in Leigh, Lancashire, England, by diagnosis

Diagnosis	Total			Males			Females		
	Days disabled since birth	Number changing jobs	Number totally incapacitated	Days disabled since birth	Number changing jobs	Number totally incapacitated	Days disabled since birth	Number changing jobs	Number totally incapacitated
Total	104,272	19	24	45,605	14	13	58,667	5	11
Rheumatoid arthritis	49,469	5	9	8,855	2	2	40,614	3	7
Osteo-arthrosis	16,030	2	3	10,283	2	2	5,747	-	1
Disk disease	14,238	6	4	11,753	5	4	2,485	1	-
Spondylitis	5,278	-	1	5,278	-	1	-	-	-
Other rheumatism	13,482	2	4	6,636	2	2	6,846	-	2
Undetermined	5,775	4	3	2,800	3	2	2,975	1	1

Source: Lawrence, 1965b.

tion rates by age, sex, and diagnosis. In Table 9.2 the rates for relevant diagnoses are provided by sex. Only a small fraction of the consultations for diseases of the bones and organs of movement are accounted for by the well-defined categories like 722, 723, and 735. This will not surprise anyone who has been in general practice or who has done arthritis surveys. It does, however, suggest that the data from general practice will not answer all the questions we should like to ask.

For a more complete albeit earlier picture, one can look at the data presented by Kalbak (1953) for Denmark. These are presented in Table 9.3, which gives a clear impression that rheumatoid arthritis was the principal crippler and that nonarticular rheumatism accounted for the bulk of the milder complaints treated in the outpatient department. It is, of course, clear that as our understanding of rheumatic diseases has progressed in the last twenty years, the diagnosis of nonarticular rheumatism, fibrositis, psychogenic rheumatism, lumbago, and so forth have been gradually replaced by more specific terms or by an admission that we are unable to classify the case. Because of the progressive changes in terminology that have been taking place at various rates in various countries, caution is needed in generalizing from the data in Tables 9.1 to 9.3.

Table 9.2   Consultation and patient consulting rates per 1,000 population by sex and selected diagnoses for 106 practices in England and Wales, 1955-56

Disease or condition (International classification)	Consultations			Patients consulting		
	Total	Males	Females	Total	Males	Females
All diseases and conditions	3,751.0	3,385.0	4,076.0	670.0	635.0	702.0
Gout (288)	2.5	4.3	1.0	0.8	1.2	0.4
Diseases of bones and organs of movement (720-749)	271.6	234.3	305.0	86.8	75.4	97.0
Rheumatoid arthritis (722)	36.2	17.6	52.7	4.8	2.0	7.3
Spondylitis (722.1)	0.7	0.8	0.5	0.2	0.2	0.1
Osteoarthritis (723)	40.7	27.7	52.3	11.2	7.2	14.7
Arthritis, unspecified (725)	19.8	14.1	24.9	5.9	4.1	7.5
Lumbago (726.0)	23.2	28.7	18.3	9.4	11.0	8.0
Other, muscular rheumatism (726)	55.7	52.8	58.2	26.7	24.4	28.8
Rheumatism, unspecified (727)	23.4	15.0	30.8	7.9	5.1	10.4
Osteitis deformans (731)	2.2	1.8	2.6	0.3	0.3	0.3
Internal derangement of knee (734)	1.7	3.0	0.6	0.6	1.0	0.3
Displacement of intervertebral disk (735)	18.6	23.5	14.3	5.0	5.7	4.4
Synovitis, bursitis and tenosynovitis (741-742)	23.0	24.5	21.7	10.2	10.0	10.4
Flat foot (746)	2.2	2.1	2.4	1.4	1.2	1.6
Hallux valgus and varus (747)	1.3	0.5	1.9	0.6	0.2	1.0
Other disease of bone, joint and musculoskeletal system (730-749)	18.3	18.7	17.9	7.0	6.6	7.3

Source: Logan and Cushion, 1958.

Table 9.3   Percent distribution by diagnosis in several severity categories

Diagnosis	Unable to work at least 1/3 time	Hospitalized	Outpatients
Rheumatoid arthritis	"Nearly All"	21	2
Gout	---	1	a
Osteoarthrosis	---	21	12
Other articular	---	8	4
Nonarticular rheumatism	---	49	82
Total		100	100

Source: Kalbak, 1953.

a Less than 0.5.

It is clearly a task for future research to provide more data on disability caused by rheumatic diseases, and medical care provided for them.

9.2 Overview. At this point we can look back and see that the rheumatic diseases constitute a major source of complaints in the population, are responsible for 7 to 9 percent of the cases of illness, of the days lost from work, and of the medical consultations, but are responsible for only about 1 percent of the hospitalizations. Rheumatoid arthritis is responsible for more consultations and disability in women, while disk degeneration is more of a problem for men. Rheumatoid arthritis is still a disease of unknown etiology but a theory about its genesis has been presented in order to stimulate further research. Osteoarthrosis appears to be related at least in part to the amount of use of the joint in question. The frequency of gout is a direct function of the level of uric acid in the serum, and we have seen that genetic factors and a variety of host and environmental factors can influence uric acid levels. Almost nothing is known about the factors that precipitate acute attacks of gout. The issue of the degree of relatedness of the various diseases in the collagen group is still unclear and may remain so until the respective etiologies are unraveled.

9.3 Directions for the Future. Along the way we have earmarked further tasks for epidemiologic research, particularly the need to investigate hypotheses about etiology with special emphasis on longitudinal studies of the natural history of the diseases in question. Furthermore, we have repeatedly observed that further studies of the genetics of the connective-tissue diseases should focus on susceptibility to the group, not on single diagnostic rubrics. Finally, we have come to the conclusion that much too little is known about the disability resulting from these affections and about the extent and nature of services necessary to reduce this disability.

BIBLIOGRAPHY
INDEX

BIBLIOGRAPHY

Abramson, J. H., "On the Diagnostic Criteria of Active Rheumatoid Arthritis," *Journal of Chronic Diseases*, 20:275-290 (May 1967).

Acheson, R. M., and J. S. Lawrence, "Social Class Gradients and Serum Uric Acid in Males and Females," *British Medical Journal*, 4:65-69 (October 11, 1969).

—— and W. M. O'Brien, "Dependence of Serum Uric Acid on Hemoglobin and Other Factors in the General Population," *Lancet*, 2:777-778 (October 8, 1966*a*).

—— —— letter to the editor, *Lancet*, 2:1320 (December 10, 1966*b*).

Adler, Emil, and J. H. Abramson, "The Use of Questions as an Indicator of Active Rheumatoid Arthritis," *Israel Journal of Medical Sciences*, 4:210-217 (March-April 1968).

—— Z. Elkan, S. Ben Hador, and R. Goldberg, "Rheumatoid Arthritis in a Jerusalem Population: I. Epidemiology of the Disease," *American Journal of Epidemiology*, 85:365-377 (May 1967*a*).

—— —— R. Goldberg, Z. Elkan, and S. Ben Hador, "Rheumatoid Arthritis in a Jerusalem Population: II. Epidemiology of Rheumatoid Factors," *American Journal of Epidemiology*, 85:378-386 (May 1967*b*).

Aho, K., H. Jalkanen, Veiko Laine, N. Ripatti, and Od Wager, "Clinical Evaluation of the Serological Tests in Rheumatoid Arthritis: I. Normal Series Collected by Random Sampling," *Acta Rheumatologica Scandinavica*, 7:201-208 (1961).

Alper, Carl, and Joseph Seitchik, "Comparison of the Archibald-Kern and Stransky Colorimetric Procedure and the Praetorius Enzymatic Procedure for the Determination of Uric Acid," *Clinical Chemistry*, 3:95-101 (April 1957).

American Rheumatism Association, "Primer on the Rheumatic Diseases," *Journal of the American Medical Association*, 190:127–140 (October 12, 1964); 425-444 (November 2, 1964); 509-530 (November 9, 1964); 741-751 (November 23, 1964).

Anderson, J. A. D., and J. J. R. Duthie, "Rheumatic Complaints in Dockyard Workers," *Annals of the Rheumatic Diseases*, 22:401-409 (November 1963).

—— —— and B. P. Moody, "Social and Economic Effects of Rheumatic Diseases in a Mining Population," *Annals of the Rheumatic Diseases*, 21:342-352 (December 1962).

Ansell, B. M., and E. G. L. Bywaters, "Rheumatoid Arthritis (Still's Disease)," *Pediatric Clinics of North America*, 10:921-939 (November 1963).

—— and J. S. Lawrence, "A Family Study in Lupus Erythematosus" (abstract), *Arthritis and Rheumatism*, 6:260 (June 1963).

—— —— "Fluoridation and the Rheumatic Diseases: A Comparison of Watford and Leigh," *Annals of the Rheumatic Diseases*, 25:67-75 (January 1965).

—— E. G. L. Bywaters, and J. S. Lawrence, "Family Studies in Still's Disease (Juvenile RA)," in P. H. Bennett and P. H. N. Wood, eds., *Population Studies of the Rheumatic Diseases* (Amsterdam: Excerpta Medica, 1968), pp. 229-234.

Armstrong, R., "Family Osteoarthritis," *Proceedings of the Royal Society of Medicine*, 13:24-29 (1920).

Atlas of Standard Radiographs of Arthritis, Epidemiology of Chronic Rheumatism, (Oxford: Blackwell, 1963), vol. 2.

Atwater, E. C., and R. F. Jacox, "The Death Certificate in Rheumatoid Arthritis," *Arthritis and Rheumatism*, 10:259 (March 1967).

Avnet, Helen, *Physician Service Patterns and Illness Rates* (New York: Group Health Insurance, Inc., 1967).

Bachman, D. M., "Survey of Rheumatoid Arthritis in Oregon" (abstract), *Arthritis and Rheumatism*, 6:761 (November 1963).

Ball, John, "Postmortem Findings in Rheumatoid Arthritis," in J. J. R. Duthie and W. R. M. Alexander, eds., *Rheumatic Disease* (Edinburgh: Edinburgh University Press — Pfizer Medical Monographs 3, 1968), p. 123.

—— and J. S. Lawrence, "Epidemiology of the Sheep Cell Agglutination Test," *Annals of the Rheumatic Diseases*, 20:235-243 (September 1961).

—— —— "The Relationship of Rheumatoid Serum Factor to Rheumatoid Arthritis: A Five Year Follow Up of a Population Sample," *Annals of the Rheumatic Diseases*, 22:311-318 (September 1963).

—— Robbert de Graaff, H. A. Valkenburg, and F. W. Boerma, "Comparative Studies of Serologic Tests for Rheumatoid Disease: I. A Comparison of a Latex Test and Two Erythrocyte Agglutination Tests in a Random Population Sample," *Arthritis and Rheumatism*, 5:55-60 (February 1962a).

—— K. J. Bloch, T. A. Burch, J. H. Kellgren, J. S. Lawrence, and V. Tsigalidou, "Comparative Studies of Serologic Tests for Rheumatoid Disease: II. A Comparison of the Bentonite Flocculation Test and the Sensitized Sheep Cell Agglutination Test," *Arthritis and Rheumatism*, 5:61-69 (February 1962b).

Barkin, R. E., "The Clinical Course of Juvenile Rheumatoid Arthritis," *Bulletin on Rheumatic Diseases*, 3:19-20 (September 1952).

Barlow, J. S., "Comparative Geography of Rheumatic Fever and Rheumatic Heart Disease, Multiple Sclerosis, and Rheumatoid Arthritis," *Journal of Chronic Diseases*, 21:265-279 (July 1968).

Barnett, E. V., Piero Balduzzi, J. H. Vaughan, and H. R. Morgan, "Search for Infectious Agents in Rheumatoid Arthritis," *Arthritis and Rheumatism*, 9:720-724 (October 1966).

Barrie, Herbert, Cedric Carter, and John Sutcliffe, "Multiple Epiphysical Dysplasia," *British Medical Journal*, 2:133-137 (July 19, 1958).

Barrow, J. F., and E. L. Armstrong, "Intestinal Protozoa and Chronic Diseases, with Special Reference to Chronic Arthritis," *Journal of the Iowa State Medical Society*, 15:553-558 (1925).

Bauer, Walter, and W. S. Clark, "The Systemic Manifestations of Rheumatoid Arthritis," *Transactions of the Association of American Physicians*, 61:339-342 (1948).

Beall, Geoffrey, and Sidney Cobb, "The Frequency Distribution of Episodes of Rheumatoid Arthritis as Shown by Periodic Examination," *Journal of Chronic Diseases*, 14:291-310 (September 1961).

Behrend, Von T., "Epidemiologische Untersuchungen über chronisch entzündliche Rheumatismusfolgen in der Bevolkerung und in Arthritiker-Familien," *Zeitschrift für Rheumaforschung*, 22:379-398 (October 1963).

Beitzke, H., "Ueber die sogen. Arthritis Deformans Atrophica," *Zeitschrift für Klinische Medizin*, 74:215-229 (1912).

Bennett, G. A., Hans Waine, and Walter Bauer, *Changes in the Knee Joint at Various Ages* (New York: The Commonwealth Fund, 1942).

Bennett, P. H., and T. A. Burch, "New York Symposium on Population Studies in the Rheumatic Diseases: New Diagnostic Criteria," *Bulletin on the Rheumatic Diseases*, 17:453-458 (April 1967).

—— —— "Rheumatoid Factor in the Blackfeet and Pima Indians," in P. H. Bennett and P. H. N. Wood, eds., *Population Studies of the Rheumatic Diseases* (Amsterdam: Excerpta Medica, 1968a), pp. 192-202.

——— ——— "The Distribution of Rheumatoid Factor and Rheumatoid Arthritis in the Families of Blackfeet and Pima Indians," *Arthritis and Rheumatism*, 11:546-553 (August 1968*b*).

——— ——— "The Genetics of Rheumatoid Arthritis," in P. H. Bennett and P. H. N. Wood, eds., *Population Studies of the Rheumatic Diseases* (Amsterdam: Excerpta Medica, 1968*c*), pp. 136-147.

——— ——— "The Epidemiologic Diagnosis of Ankylosing Spondylitis," in P. H. Bennett and P. H. N. Wood, eds., *Population Studies of the Rheumatic Diseases* (Amsterdam: Excerpta Medica, 1968*d*), pp. 305-313.

——— ——— "Serum Uric Acid and Gout in Blackfeet and Pima Indians," in P. H. Bennett and P. H. N. Wood, eds., *Population Studies of the Rheumatic Diseases* (Amsterdam: Excerpta Medica, 1968*e*), pp. 358-364.

——— and P. H. N. Wood, eds., *Population Studies of the Rheumatic Diseases* (Amsterdam: Excerpta Medica, 1968).

Berens, D. L., Rukan Lin, B. M. Norcross, and L. M. Lookie, "Early Recognition of Adult Rheumatoid Arthritis (Roentgen Findings)" (abstract), *Arthritis and Rheumatism*, 11:467 (June 1968).

Berglöf, F.-E., "Arthritis and Intestinal Infection," *Acta Rheumatologica Scandinavica*, 9:141-149 (1963).

Berkson, Joseph, "Limitations of the Application of Fourfold Table Analysis to Hospital Data," *Biometrics Bulletin*, 2:47-53 (June 1946).

——— "Mortality and Marital Status: Reflections on the Derivation of Etiology from Statistics," *American Journal of Public Health*, 52:1318-1329 (August 1962).

Black, J. A., H. E. Lewis, C. K. M. Thacker, and A. K. Thould, "Tristan da Cunha: General Medical Investigations," *British Medical Journal*, 2:1018-1024 (October 26, 1963).

Blauch, M. B., and F. C. Koch, "A New Method for the Determination of Uric Acid in Blood, with Uricase," *Journal of Biological Chemistry*, 130:443-454 (October 1939).

Blom, G. E., and B. Whipple, "A Method of Studying Emotional Factors in Children with Rheumatoid Arthritis," in Lucy Jessner and Eleanor Pavenstedt, eds., *Dynamic Psychopathology in Childhood* (New York: Grune and Stratton, 1959).

Blumberg, B. S., "Genetics and Rheumatoid Arthritis," *Arthritis and Rheumatism*, 3:178-185 (April 1960).

——— K. J. Bloch, R. L. Black, and Charles Dotter, "A Study of the Prevalence of Arthritis in Alaskan Eskimos," *Arthritis and Rheumatism*, 4:325-341 (August 1961).

Blumberg, Baruch, and Charles Ragan, "The Natural History of Rheumatoid Spondylitis," *Medicine*, 35:1-31 (February 1956).

Boyle, J. A., W. R. Greig, M. K. Jasani, Anne Duncan, Michael Diver, and W. W. Buchanan, "Relative Rates of Genetic and Environmental Factors in the Control of Serum Uric Acid Levels in Normouricaemic Subjects," *Annals of the Rheumatic Diseases*, 26:234-238 (May 1967).

Bremner, J. M., and J. S. Lawrence, "Population Studies of Serum Uric Acid," *Proceedings of the Royal Society of Medicine*, 59:319-325 (April 1966).

——— ——— and W. E. Miall, "Degenerative Joint Disease in a Jamaican Rural Population," *Annals of the Rheumatic Diseases*, 27:326-332 (July 1968).

Britten, R. H., S. D. Collins, and J. J. Fitzgerald, "The National Health Survey: Some General Findings as to Disease, Accidents, and Impairments in Urban Areas," *Public Health Reports*, 55:444-470 (March 15, 1940).

Brøchner-Mortensen, Knud, Sidney Cobb, and B. S. Rose, "Report of Sub-Committee on Criteria for the Diagnosis of Gout in Surveys," in M. R.

Jeffrey and John Ball, eds., *The Epidemiology of Chronic Rheumatism* (Oxford: Blackwell, 1963), vol. 1, pp. 295-297.

Brooks, G. W., and Sidney Cobb, "Studies in Latex Agglutination: An Approach to the Determination of Optimum Conditions for Discrimination between Rheumatoids and Normals," *Arthritis and Rheumatism*, 6:198-207 (June 1963).

—— —— "Rheumatoid Factors: Ubiquity and Specificity," *Rheumatism* (London), 20:43-50 (April 1964).

—— and Ernst Mueller, "Serum Urate Concentrations in University Professors: Relation to Drive, Achievement and Leadership," *Journal of the American Medical Association*, 195:415-418 (February 7, 1966).

Brown, A. R., and B. S. Rose, "Familial Precocious Polyarticular Osteoarthrosis of Chrondrodysplastic Type," *New Zealand Medical Journal*, 65:449-461 (July 1966).

Brown, Robert, and Claire Lingg, "Musculoskeletal Complaints in an Industry: Annual Complaint Rate and Diagnosis, Absenteeism and Economic Loss," *Arthritis and Rheumatism*, 4:283-302 (June 1961).

Burbank, R., "Arthritis through the Ages," *Tri-State Medical Journal*, 15:2903-2911 (March 1943).

Burch, T. A., personal communication, 1964.

—— personal communication, June 6, 1967.

—— "Mortality from Rheumatoid Arthritis in the United States, 1959-1961," in P. H. Bennett and P. H. N. Wood, eds., *Population Studies of the Rheumatic Diseases* (Amsterdam: Excerpta Medica, 1968), pp. 39-42.

—— J. J. Bunim, and K. J. Bloch, "Studies in Relatives of Patients with Sjögren's Syndrome," in M. R. Jeffrey and John Ball, eds., *The Epidemiology of Chronic Rheumatism* (Oxford: Blackwell, 1963), vol. 1, pp. 267-276.

—— W. M. O'Brien, Richard Need, and L. T. Kurland, "Hyperuricemia and Gout in the Mariana Islands," *Annals of the Rheumatic Diseases*, 25:114-116 (May 1966).

Bywaters, E. G. L., "Family Studies of Rheumatoid Arthritis and Lupus Erythematosus in Great Britain," in M. R. Jeffrey and John Ball, eds., *The Epidemiology of Chronic Rheumatism* (Oxford: Blackwell, 1963), vol. 1, pp. 249-257.

—— "Heberden Oration, 1966: Categorization in Medicine: A Survey of Still's Disease," *Annals of the Rheumatic Diseases*, 26:185-192 (May 1967).

—— "Diagnostic Criteria for Still's Disease (Juvenile RA)," in P. H. Bennett and P. H. N. Wood, eds., *Population Studies of the Rheumatic Diseases* (Amsterdam: Excerpta Medica, 1968), pp. 235-240.

—— and B. M. Ansell, "Sacroiliitis in Juvenile Chronic Polyarthritis," *Zeitschrift für Rheumaforschung*, 24:122-125 (summer 1965).

—— and V. P. Holloway, "Measurement of Serum Uric Acid in Great Britain in 1963," *Annals of the Rheumatic Diseases*, 23:236-239 (May 1964).

Calabro, J. J., and J. M. Marchesano, "Current Concepts: Juvenile Rheumatoid Arthritis," *New England Journal of Medicine*, 277:696-699 (September 28, 1967); 746-749 (October 5, 1967).

—— —— "The Early Natural History of Juvenile Rheumatoid Arthritis: A 10-Year Follow-up Study of 100 Cases," *Medical Clinics of North America*, 52:567-591 (May 1968).

Canada, Bureau of Statistics, *Illness and Health Care in Canada: Canadian Sickness Survey 1950-51* (Ottawa: Queens Printer, 1960).

Caplan, P. S., L. M. Freedman, and T. P. Connelly, "Degenerative Joint Disease of the Lumbar Spine in Coal Miners: A Clinical and X-ray Study," *Arthritis and Rheumatism*, 9:693-702 (October 1966).

Carroll, R. E., and William Haddon, Jr., "Pitfalls in the Use of 'Accident' Victims as Comparison Groups," *Journal of Chronic Diseases*, 18:601-603 (July 1965).

Case, R. A. M., "Cohort Analysis of Mortality Rates as an Historical or Narrative Technique," *British Journal of Preventive and Social Medicine*, 10:159-171 (October 1956).

Cathcart, E. S., J. A. Bolzan, and J. B. O'Sullivan, "Patterns of Radiologic Abnormalities in the Hands Related to Rheumatoid Arthritis," in P. H. Bennett and P. H. N. Wood, eds., *Population Studies of the Rheumatic Diseases* (Amsterdam: Excerpta Medica, 1968), pp. 423-434.

Catterall, R. D., "Uveitis Arthritis and Non-Specific Genital Infection," *British Journal of Venereal Disease*, 36:27-29 (March 1960).

Chen, Edith, and Sidney Cobb, "Family Structure in Relation to Health and Disease," *Journal of Chronic Diseases*, 12:544-567 (November 1960).

Cleveland, S. E., E. E. Reitman, and E. J. Brewer, Jr., "Psychological Factors in Juvenile Rheumatoid Arthritis," *Arthritis and Rheumatism*, 8:1152-1158 (December 1965).

Coates, V., and L. Delicati, "The Correlation between Certain Rheumatic Diseases and Occupation," *Acta Rheumatologica*, 4:28–32 (December 1932).

Cobb, Sidney, unpublished progress report, 1956.

—— "Contained Hostility in Rheumatoid Arthritis," *Arthritis and Rheumatism*, 2:419-425 (October 1959).

—— "On the Development of Diagnostic Criteria," *Arthritis and Rheumatism*, 3:91-95 (February 1960).

—— "A Method for the Epidemiologic Study of Remittent Disease," *American Journal of Public Health*, 52:1119-1125 (July 1962).

—— "Hyperuricemia in Executives," in M. R. Jeffrey and John Ball, eds., *The Epidemiology of Chronic Rheumatism* (Oxford: Blackwell, 1963), vol. 1, pp. 182-196.

—— "The Epidemiology of Rheumatoid Arthritis," *Arthritis and Rheumatism*, 8:76-79 (February 1965*a*).

—— "The Prevention of Gout," *American Journal of Public Health*, 55:353-354 (March 1965*b*).

—— and William Hall, "A Newly Identified Cluster of Diseases: Rheumatoid Arthritis, Peptic Ulcer and Tuberculosis," *Journal of the American Medical Association*, 193:1077-1079 (September 27, 1965).

—— and S. V. Kasl, "The Epidemiology of Rheumatoid Arthritis," *American Journal of Public Health*, 56:1657-1663 (October 1966).

—— —— "Epidemiologic Contributions to the Etiology of Rheumatoid Arthritis, with Special Attention to Psychological and Social Factors," in P. H. Bennett and P. H. N. Wood, eds., *Population Studies of the Rheumatic Diseases* (Amsterdam: Excerpta Medica, 1968), pp. 75-82.

—— and J. S. Lawrence, "Towards a Geography of Rheumatoid Arthritis," *Bulletin on the Rheumatic Diseases*, 7:133-134 (April 1957).

—— Florence Anderson, and Walter Bauer, "Length of Life and Cause of Death in Rheumatoid Arthritis," *New England Journal of Medicine*, 249:553-556 (October 1953).

—— W. R. Merchant, and J. E. Warren, "An Epidemiologic Look at the Problem of Classification in the Field of Arthritis," *Journal of Chronic Diseases*, 2:50-54 (July 1955).

—— D. J. Thompson, Joseph Rosenbaum, J. E. Warren, and W. R. Merchant, "On the Measurement of the Prevalence of Arthritis and Rheumatism from Interview Data," *Journal of Chronic Diseases*, 3:134-139 (February 1956).

—— W. R. Merchant, and Theodore Rubin, "The Relation of Symptoms to Osteoarthritis," *Journal of Chronic Diseases*, 5:197-204 (February 1957*a*).

—— J. E. Warren, W. R. Merchant, and D. J. Thompson, "An Estimate of the Prevalence of Rheumatoid Arthritis," *Journal of Chronic Diseases*, 5:636-643 (June 1957*b*).

—— Martha Miller, and Martha Wieland, "On the Relationship between Divorce and Rheumatoid Arthritis," *Arthritis and Rheumatism*, 2:414-418 (October 1959).

—— S. V. Kasl, Edith Chen, and Roger Christenfeld, "Some Psychological and Social Characteristics of Patients Hospitalized for Rheumatoid Arthritis, Hypertension, and Duodenal Ulcer," *Journal of Chronic Diseases*, 18:1259-1278 (December 1965).

—— G. W. Brooks, and S. V. Kasl, "Serum Uric Acid Levels," *Lancet*, 2:1320 (December 10, 1966*a*).

—— —— —— and W. E. Connelly, "The Health of People Changing Jobs: A Description of a Longitudinal Study," *American Journal of Public Health*, 56:1476-1481 (September 1966*b*).

—— Patricia Hunt, and Ernest Harburg, "The Intrafamilial Transmission of Rheumatoid Arthritis: II. An Interview Measure of Rheumatoid Arthritis," *Journal of Chronic Diseases*, 22:203-216 (September 1969*a*).

—— S. V. Kasl, J. R. P. French, Jr., Guttorm Nörstebö, "The Intrafamilial Transmission of Rheumatoid Arthritis: VII. Why Do Wives with Rheumatoid Arthritis have Husbands with Peptic Ulcer?" *Journal of Chronic Diseases*, 22:279-294 (September 1969*b*).

—— Walter Bauer, and Isabel Whiting, "Environmental Factors in Rheumatoid Arthritis: A Study of the Relationship between the Onset and Exacerbations of Arthritis and the Emotional or Environmental Factor," *Journal of the American Medical Association*, 113:668-670 (August 19, 1939).

Collins, D. H., "Osteoarthritis," *Journal of Bone and Joint Surgery* (Britain), 35B:518-520 (November 1953).

Collins, S. D., "Frequency and Volume of Doctors' Calls Among Males and Females in 9,000 Families, Based on Nationwide Periodic Canvasses, 1928-31," *Public Health Reports*, 55:1977-2020 (November 1, 1940).

Commission on Chronic Illness, *Chronic Illness in the United States: IV. Chronic Illness in a Large City: The Baltimore Study* (Cambridge, Mass.: Harvard University Press, 1957).

Copeman, W. S. C., *Textbook of the Rheumatic Diseases*, 3rd ed. (Edinburgh: Livingstone, 1964).

Crain, D. C., "Interphalangeal Osteoarthritis: Characterized by Painful Inflammatory Episodes Resulting in Deformity of the Proximal and Distal Articulations," *Journal of the American Medical Association*, 175:1049-1053 (March 25, 1961).

Cowdrey, S. C., "Hyperuricemia in Infectious Mononucleosis," *Journal of the American Medical Association*, 196:319-321 (April 1966).

Danichewsky, G., *Le Rheumatisme et le Travail Professionel* (Moscow, 1932, Opus Cit. by E. T. Coneybeare and J. A. Glover, *Rheumatism in Relation to Industry: A Survey of Chronic Rheumatic Diseases* (Oxford: Oxford University Press, 1938).

Das Gupta, S. C., "Genesis of Gout: Its Relation to Blood Pressure and Antagonism to Tuberculosis," *Indian Medical Record*, 55:97-105 (April 1935).

Dawber, T. R., P. E. Barry, and A. P. Hall, "Uric Acid, Gout and Coronary Heart Disease: Observations from the Framingham Heart Study," paper read before the 92nd annual meeting of the American Public Health Association, October 9, 1964.

de Blécourt, J. J., and A. H. M. Basart, *Investigation as to the Prevalence of Rheumatic Diseases and to their Dependence on the Degree of Dampness in Dwellings*, Research Institute for Public Health Engineering T.N.O. report no. 20, Netherlands, December 1953.

—— A. Polman, and T. de Blécourt-Meindersma, "Hereditary Factors in Rheumatoid Arthritis and Ankylosing Spondylitis," *Annals of the Rheumatic Diseases*, 20:215-223 (September 1961).

Decker, J. L., ed., *Proceedings of the Conference on the Relationship of Mycoplasma to Rheumatoid Arthritis and Related Diseases*, PHS pub. no. 1523 (Washington, D.C.: Public Health Service, 1966).

—— and J. J. Lane, "Gouty Arthritis in Filipinos," *New England Journal of Medicine*, 261:805–806 (October 15, 1959).

—— —— and W. E. Reynolds, "Hyperuricemia in a Male Filipino Population," *Arthritis and Rheumatism*, 5:144-155 (April 1962).

de Forest, G. K., M. B. Mucci, and P. L. Boisvert, "Two-Year Comparative Study of Serial Hemagglutination Tests Done on Groups of Rheumatoid Arthritis Patients," *Arthritis and Rheumatism*, 1:387-391 (October 1958).

de Graaff, Robbert, *De Reumatoide Arthritis in Nederland* (Proefschrift Rijksuniversiteit te Leiden, Assen: Van Gorcum, 1962).

—— V. A. I. Laine, and J. S. Lawrence, "Comparison of Surveys in Various Northern European Countries," in M. R. Jeffrey and John Ball, eds., *The Epidemiology of Chronic Rheumatism* (Oxford: Blackwell, 1963), vol. 1, pp. 228-238.

Demartini, F. E., "Hyperuricemia Induced by Drugs," *Arthritis and Rheumatism*, 8:823-829 (October 1965).

den Ousten, S. A., personal communication at the Third International Symposium on Population Studies of the Rheumatic Diseases, June 5-10, 1966.

Densen, P. M., personal communication, October 3, 1956.

—— C. A. D'Alonzo, and M. G. Mann, "Opportunities and Problems in the Study of Chronic Disease in Industry," *Journal of Chronic Diseases*, 1:231-252 (March 1955).

Dodge, H. J., personal communication, June 1964.

—— and W. M. Mikkelsen, "The Relationship of Serum Uric Acid Scores to Occupation, Smoking and Drinking Habits in Tecumseh, Mich., 1959-60," paper read before the 92nd annual meeting of the American Public Health Association, October 9, 1964.

Dorn, H. F., and I. M. Moriyama, "Uses and Significance of Multiple Cause Tabulations for Mortality Statistics," *American Journal of Public Health*, 54:400-406 (March 1964).

Dorpat, T. L., W. F. Anderson, and H. S. Ripley, "The Relationship of Physical Illness to Suicide," in H. L. P. Resnik, ed., *Suicidal Behaviors: Diagnosis and Management* (Boston: Little, Brown & Co., 1968), pp. 209-219.

Dresner, Ellis, "Aetiology and Pathogenesis of Rheumatoid Arthritis," *American Journal of Medicine*, 18:74-111 (January 1955).

Dreyfuss, F., and P. Hamosh, "A Coronary Disease Study Among Cochin Jews in Israel," *American Journal of Medical Sciences*, 240:769-775 (December 1960).

—— P. Hamosh, Y. G. Adam, and B. Kallner, "Coronary Heart Disease and Hypertension Among Jews Immigrated to Israel from the Atlas Mountain

Region of North Africa," *American Heart Journal*, 62:470-477 (October 1961).

—— Elisheva Yaron, and Miriam Balogh, "Blood Uric Acid Levels in Various Ethnic Groups in Israel," *American Journal of the Medical Sciences*, 247:438-444 (April 1964).

Dubois, E. L., *Lupus Erythematosus: A Review of the Current Studies of Discoid and Systemic Lupus Erythematosus and their Variants* (New York: McGraw-Hill, 1966).

Duff, I. F., W. M. Mikkelsen, H. J. Dodge, and D. S. Himes, "Comparison of Uric Acid Levels in Some Oriental and Caucasian Groups Unselected as to Gout or Hyperuricemia," *Arthritis and Rheumatism*, 11:184-190 (April 1968).

Duncan, H., and A. St.J. Dixon, "Gout, Familial Hyperuricemia, and Renal Disease," *Quarterly Journal of Medicine*, New Series 29:127-135 (January 1960).

Dunn, J. P., G. W. Brooks, Judith Mausner, G. P. Rodnan, and Sidney Cobb, "Social Class Gradient of Serum Uric Acid Levels in Males," *Journal of the American Medical Association*, 185:431-436 (August 10, 1963).

Duthie, J. J. R., P. E. Brown, L. H. Truelove, F. D. Baragar, and A. J. Lawrie, "Course and Prognosis in Rheumatoid Arthritis," *Annals of the Rheumatic Diseases*, 23:193-204 (May 1964).

Edström, Gunnar, "Klinische Studien über den Chronischen Gelenkrheumatismus, das Erbbild," *Acta Medica Scandinavica*, 108:398-413 (1941).

—— "Rheumatism a Public Health Problem in Sweden: Field Studies of Population in Certain Districts during Summer of 1943," *Upsala Läkareförenings Förhandligar N.F.*, 49:303-358 (1944).

Ehrström, M. C., "Medical Studies in North Greenland, 1948-1949: V. Rheumatic Diseases. Comparative Investigations of the Incidence," *Acta Medica Scandinavica*, 140:412-415 (1951).

Emery, A. E. H., and J. S. Lawrence, "Genetics of Ankylosing Spondylitis," *Journal of Medical Genetics*, 4:239-244 (December 1967).

Emmerson, B. T., "Heredity in Primary Gout," *Australasian Annals of Medicine*, 9:168-175 (August 1960).

Epstein, F. H., Thomas Francis, Jr., N. S. Hayner, B. C. Johnson, M. O. Kjelsberg, J. A. Napier, L. D. Ostrander, Jr., M. W. Payne, and H. J. Dodge, "Prevalence of Chronic Diseases and Distribution of Selected Physiologic Variables in a Total Community, Tecumseh, Michigan," *American Journal of Epidemiology*, 81:307-322 (May 1965).

Erasmus, D. D., "Scleroderma in Gold Miners on the Witwatersrand with Particular Reference to Pulmonary Manifestations," *South African Journal of Laboratory and Clinical Medicine*, 3:209-231 (September 1957).

Etter, L. E., J. P. Dunn, A. G. Kammer, L. H. Asmond, and L. C. Reese, "Gastroduodenal X-ray Diagnosis: A Comparison of Radiographic Techniques and Interpretations," *Radiology*, 74:766-770 (May 1960).

Eve, F. S., "Bones of Ancient Egyptians Showing Periostitis Associated with Osteo-arthritis and Symmetrical Senile Atrophy of the Skull," *Transactions of the Pathological Society of London*, 41:242-248 (1890).

Faires, J. S., and D. J. McCarty, "Acute Arthritis in Man and Dog After Intrasynovial Injection of Sodium Urate Crystals," *Lancet*, 2:682–685 (October 6, 1962).

Fisher, H. W., "The Diseases of Filipino Men," *Hawaii Medical Journal*, 18:252-254 (January-February 1959).

Folin, O., and W. Denis, "A New (Colorimetric) Method for the Determination of Uric Acid in Blood," *Journal of Biological Chemistry*, 13:469-475 (January 1913).

Ford, D. K., "Evidence for an Infectious Etiology of Rheumatoid Arthritis," *Medical Clinics of North America*, 52:673-676 (May 1968).

—— and A. M. deMos, "Serum Uric Acid Levels of Healthy Caucasian, Chinese and Haida Indian Males in British Columbia," *Canadian Medical Association Journal*, 90:1295-1297 (June 6, 1964).

Francis, Thomas, Jr., and F. H. Epstein, "Survey Methods in General Populations: Studies of a Total Community, Tecumseh, Michigan," *Milbank Memorial Fund Quarterly*, 43:333-342 (April 1965).

Francon, F., "Extensive Form of Hypertrophic Arthritis," *Rheumatism* (London), 6:17-19 (January 1950).

French, J. G., H. J. Dodge, M. O. Kjelsberg, W. M. Mikkelsen, and W. J. Schull, "A Study of Familial Aggregation of Serum Uric Acid Levels in the Population of Tecumseh, Michigan, 1959-1960," *American Journal of Epidemiology*, 86:214-224 (January 1967).

Funkenstein, D. H., "Psychophysiological Relationship of Asthma and Urticaria to Mental Illness," *Psychosomatic Medicine*, 12:377-385 (November-December 1950).

Garrod, A. B., "Observations on Certain Pathological Conditions of the Blood and Urine in Gout, Rheumatism and Bright's Disease," *Medico-Chirurgical Transactions*, Royal Medical and Chirurgical Society of London, 31:83-97 (1848).

Garrod, A. E., *Treatise on Rheumatism and Rheumatoid Arthritis* (London: Charles Griffin, 1890).

Gauchat, R. D., personal communication, March 20, 1957.

Geist, Harold, *The Psychological Aspects of Rheumatoid Arthritis* (Springfield, Ill.: Charles C. Thomas, 1966).

Gjørup, S., H. E. Poulsen, and E. Praetorius, "The Uric Acid Concentration in Serum Determined by Enzymatic Spectrophotometry," *Scandinavian Journal of Clinical and Laboratory Medicine*, 7:201-203 (1955).

Glover, J. A., "Milroy Lectures on the Incidence of Rheumatic Diseases: II. Rheumatism in Industry," *Lancet*, 1:607-612 (March 22, 1930); "III. Incidence of Chronic Arthritis," *Lancet* 1:733-738 (April 5, 1930).

Glyn, J. H., I. Sutherland, G. F. Walker, and A. C. Young, "Low Incidence of Osteoarthrosis in Hip and Knee after Anterior Poliomyelitis: A Late Review," *British Medical Journal*, 2:739-742 (September 24, 1966).

Gofton, J. P., tables given to the author at the Third International Symposium, New York, June 1966, in connection with the discussion reported on page 298 of Bennett and Wood (1968).

—— H. S. Robinson, and G. E. Price, "A Study of Rheumatic Disease in a Canadian Indian Population: II. Rheumatoid Arthritis in the Haida Indians," *Annals of the Rheumatic Diseases*, 23:364-371 (September 1964).

—— J. S. Lawrence, P. H. Bennett, and T. A. Burch, "Sacroiliitis in Eight Populations," *Annals of the Rheumatic Diseases*, 25:528-533 (November 1966).

Goldman, Franz, "Patients in Clinic Disease Hospitals: A Profile," *American Journal of Public Health*, 52:646-655 (April 1962).

Good, A. E., "Reiter's Disease and Ankylosing Spondylitis," *Acta Rheumatologica Scandinavica*, 11:305-317 (Fascicle 4, 1965).

Gordon, J. E., "The Newer Epidemiology," in *Tomorrow's Horizon in Public Health: Transactions of the 1950 Conference of the Public Health Association of New York City, New York* (Public Health Association of New York City, 1950).

Gregg, D., "Paucity of Arthritis among Psychotic Cases," *American Journal of Psychiatry*, 95:853-858 (January 1939).

Grokoest, A. W., A. I. Snyder, and Ralph Schlaeger, *Juvenile Rheumatoid Arthritis* (Boston: Little, Brown & Co., 1962).

Gruber, G. B., "Zur Frage der Periarteritis Nodosa, mit Besonderer Berücksichtigung der Gallenblasen- und Nieren-Beteiligung," *Virchow's Archiv für Pathologische Anatomic*, 258:441-501 (1925).

Haenszel, William, D. B. Loveland, and M. G. Sirken, "Lung-cancer Mortality as Related to Residence and Smoking Histories: I. White Males," *Journal of the National Cancer Institute*, 28:947-1001 (April 1962).

Hailman, D. E., "Health Status of Adults in the Productive Ages," *Public Health Reports*, 56:2071-2087 (October 24, 1941).

Hall, A. P., personal communication, October 1963.

—— P. E. Barry, and T. R. Dawber, "The Relationship between Hyperuricemia and Gouty Arthritis and the Risk of Developing Coronary Heart Disease" (abstract), *Arthritis and Rheumatism*, 7:312 (June 1964).

—— —— —— and P. M. McNamara, "Epidemiology of Gout and Hyperuricemia: A Long-Term Population Study," *American Journal of Medicine*, 42:27-37 (January 1967).

Harburg, Ernest, S. V. Kasl, Joyce Tabor, and Sidney Cobb, "Intrafamilial Transmission of Rheumatoid Arthritis: IV. Recalled Parent-Child Relations by Rheumatoid Arthritis and Controls," *Journal of Chronic Diseases*, 22:223-238 (September 1969).

Hartmann, F., T. Behrend, H. Deicher, R. Fricke, H. Manecke, and G. Walpurger, "Studies in Germany," in M. R. Jeffrey and John Ball, eds., *The Epidemiology of Chronic Rheumatism* (Oxford: Blackwell, 1963), vol. 1, pp. 277–286.

Hartung, E. F., "Historical Considerations," *Metabolism: Clinical and Experimental*, 6:196-208 (May 1957).

Hauge, M., and B. Harvald, "Heredity in Gout and Hyperuricemia," *Acta Medica Scandinavica*, 152:247-257 (1955).

Healey, L. A., Jr., J. E. Z. Caner, and J. L. Decker, "Ethnic Variations in Serum Uric Acid: I. Filipino Hyperuricemia in a Controlled Environment," *Arthritis and Rheumatism*, 9:288-294 (April 1966).

Health Insurance Plan Statistical Report (New York: Health Insurance Plan of Greater New York, Division of Research and Statistics, 1961).

Heine, J., "Uber die Arthritis Deformans," *Virchow's Archiv für Pathologic, Anatomic und Physiologic*, 260:521-663 (April 1926).

Hermann, R., "Uber die Erblichkeit bei der Arthrosis Degenerativa," *Zeitschrift für Menschliche Vererbungs- und Konstitutionslehre*, 19:707-720 (May 1936).

Hollander, J. L., E. M. Brown, Jr., R. A. Jessar, Klaus Hummeler, and Werner Henle, "Studies on the Relationship of Virus Infections to Early or Acute Rheumatoid Arthritis," *Archives of Interamerican Rheumatism*, 5:137-157 (June 1962).

Holsti, Ö., and A. S. Huuskonen, "Heredo-familial Arthritis: Study of 4 Generations of Arthritis-Family," *Acta Medica Scandinavica*, suppl. 89:128-138 (1938).

—— and V. Rantasalo, "On the Occurrence of Arthritis in Finland," *Acta Medica Scandinavica*, 88:180-195 (1936).

Hormell, R. S., "Notes on the History of Rheumatism and Gout," *New England Journal of Medicine*, 223:754-760 (November 7, 1940).

Horvath, W. J., "The Effect of Physician Bias in Medical Diagnosis," *Behavioral Science*, 9:334-340 (October 1964).

Houpt, J. B., M. A. Ogryzlo, M. A. Hunt, and A. A. Fletcher, "Tryptophan Metabolism and Rheumatoid Arthritis," in *Studies of Rheumatoid Disease*, Proceedings of the Third Canadian Conference on Research in the Rheumatic Diseases (Toronto: University of Toronto Press, 1966).

Ishmael, W. K., "Primary Osteoarthritis, Migraine Headaches, and Motion Sickness: Familial Interrelationship," *Journal of the American Medical Association*, 201:103-105 (July 10, 1967).

Jackson, D. S., and J. H. Kellgren, "Hyaluronic Acid in Heberden's Nodes," *Annals of the Rheumatic Diseases*, 16:238-240 (June 1957).

Jacox, R. F., Sanford Meyerowitz, and William Hess, "Monozygotic Twins Discordant for Rheumatoid Arthritis: A Genetic, Clinical and Psychological Study of Eight Sets," in P. H. Bennett and P. H. N. Wood, eds., *Population Studies of the Rheumatic Diseases* (Amsterdam: Excerpta Medica, 1968), pp. 128-135.

Jeffrey, M. R., and John Ball, eds., *The Epidemiology of Chronic Rheumatism* (Oxford: Blackwell, 1963), vol. 1.

Jensen, Julius, D. H. Blankenhorn, Philip Sturgeon, H. P. Chin, and A. G. Ware, "Serum Lipids and Serum Uric Acid in Human Twins," *Journal of Lipid Research*, 6:193-205 (April 1965).

Kahlmeter, G., "Examen Statistique des Causes d'Invalidité, fait d'après les Demandes Adressés à la Direction de Pensions de Retraite pendant l'Année 1918, sur lesquelles les Pensions Supplémentaires Furent Accordées," *Acta Medica Scandinavica*, 59:153-179 (1923).

Kahn, Robert L., and Charles F. Cannell, *The Dynamics of Interviewing* (New York: John Wiley and Sons, Inc., 1965).

Kalbak, K., "Rheumatic Diseases in Denmark," *Annals of the Rheumatic Diseases*, 12:306-309 (December 1953).

Kantor, T. G., and Martin Tanner, "Rubella Arthritis and Rheumatoid Arthritis," *Arthritis and Rheumatism*, 5:378-383 (August 1962).

Kasl, S. V., and Sidney Cobb, "Some Psychological Factors Associated with Illness Behavior and Selected Illnesses," *Journal of Chronic Diseases*, 17:325-345 (April 1964).

—— —— "Health Behavior, Illness Behavior and Sick Role Behavior," *Archives of Environmental Health*, 12:246-266 (February 1966).

—— —— "The Intrafamilial Transmission of Rheumatoid Arthritis: V. Differences Between Rheumatoid Arthritis and Controls on Selected Personality Variables," *Journal of Chronic Diseases*, 22:239-258 (September 1969*a*).

—— —— "The Intrafamilial Transmission of Rheumatoid Arthritis: VI. Association of Rheumatoid Arthritis with Several Types of Status Inconsistency," *Journal of Chronic Diseases*, 22:259-278 (September 1969*b*).

—— —— and G. W. Brooks, "Changes in Serum Uric Acid and Serum Cholesterol in Men Undergoing Job Loss," *Journal of the American Medical Association*, 206:1500-1507 (November 11, 1968).

Kay, April, and Francis Boch, "Subfertility before and after Development of Rheumatoid Arthritis in Women," *Annals of the Rheumatic Diseases*, 24:169-173 (March 1965).

Kellgren, J. H., "Radiological Signs of Rheumatoid Arthritis," *Annals of the Rheumatic Diseases*, 15:55-60 (March 1956).

—— "Osteoarthrosis in Patients and Populations," *British Medical Journal*, 2:1-6 (July 1, 1961).

—— "Diagnostic Criteria for Population Studies," *Bulletin on the Rheumatic Diseases*, 3:291-292 (November 1962).

—— "Heberden Oration, 1963: The Epidemiology of Rheumatic Diseases," *Annals of the Rheumatic Diseases*, 23:109-122 (March 1964).

—— "Clinical Rheumatoid Arthritis, Rheumatoid Factor, and Erosive Arthritis: A Critical Examination of the Inter-Relationship," in P. H. Bennett and P. H. N. Wood, eds., *Population Studies of the Rheumatic Diseases* (Amsterdam: Excerpta Medica, 1968), pp. 151-159.

—— and J. S. Lawrence, "Rheumatism in Miners, X-ray Study," *British Journal of Industrial Medicine*, 9:197-207 (July 1952).

—— —— "Rheumatoid Arthritis in a Population Sample," *Annals of the Rheumatic Diseases*, 15:1-11 (March 1956).

—— —— "Radiological Assessment of Osteoarthrosis," *Annals of the Rheumatic Diseases*, 16:494-502 (December 1957*a*).

—— —— "Radiological Assessment of Rheumatoid Arthritis,"*Annals of the Rheumatic Diseases*, 16:485-493 (December 1957*b*).

—— —— "Osteoarthrosis and Disk Degeneration in an Urban Population," *Annals of the Rheumatic Diseases*, 17:388-397 (December 1958).

—— and R. Moore, "Generalized Osteoarthritis and Heberden's Nodes," *British Medical Journal*, 1:181-187 (January 26, 1952).

—— J. S. Lawrence, and Jean Aitken-Swan, "Rheumatic Complaints in an Urban Population," *Annals of the Rheumatic Diseases*, 12:5-15 (March 1953).

—— John Ball, R. W. Fairbrother, and K. L. Barnes, "Suppurative Arthritis Complicating Rheumatoid Arthritis," *British Medical Journal*, no. 5081:1193-1200 (May 24, 1958).

—— J. S. Lawrence, and Frieda Bier, "Genetic Factors in Generalized Osteoarthritis," *Annals of the Rheumatic Diseases*, 23:109-122 (March 1964).

Kellum, R. E., and J. R. Haserick, "Systemic Lupus Erythematosus: A Statistical Evaluation of the Mortality Based on a Consecutive Series of 299 Patients," *Archives of Internal Medicine*, 113:200-207 (February 1964).

Kelly, M., "Monarticular Trauma and Rheumatoid Arthritis," *Annals of the Rheumatic Diseases*, 10:307-319 (September 1951).

Kidd, K. L., and J. B. Peter, "Erosive Osteoarthrosis," *Radiology*, 86:640-647 (April 1966).

King, S. H., "Psychosocial Factors Associated with Rheumatoid Arthritis: An Evaluation of the Literature," *Journal of Chronic Diseases*, 2:287-302 (September 1955).

—— and Sidney Cobb, "Psychosocial Factors in the Epidemiology of Rheumatoid Arthritis," *Journal of Chronic Diseases*, 7:466-475 (June 1958).

Kline, B. S., and A. M. Young, "Cases of Reversible and Irreversible Allergic Inflammation," *Journal of Allergy*, 6:258–272 (March 1935).

La Du, B. N., J. E. Seegmiller, L. Laster and V. Zannoni, "Alcaptonuria and Ochronotic Arthritis," *Bulletin on the Rheumatic Diseases*, 8:163-164 (May 1958).

Laine, V. A. I., personal communication, February 7, 1964.

Lawrence, J. S., "Communication," *Proceedings of the Royal Society of Medicine*, 53:522-526 (May 1960).

—— "Prevalence of Rheumatoid Arthritis," *Annals of the Rheumatic Diseases*, 20:11-17 (March 1961*a*).

—— "Rheumatism in Cotton Operatives," *British Journal of Industrial Medicine*, 18:270-276 (October 1961*b*).

—— "The Influence of Climate on the Prevalence of Rheumatic Complaints," *Manchester Medical Gazette*, 42:1-4 (December 1962).

—— "Surveys of Rheumatic Complaints in the Population," in A. St.J. Dixon, ed., *Progress in Clinical Rheumatology* (Boston: Little, Brown & Co., 1965*a*), pp. 1-9.

—— personal communication, July 1965*b*.

—— "Genetics of Rheumatoid Factor and Rheumatoid Arthritis," *Clinical and Experimental Immunology*, 2, suppl.:769-783 (December 1967).

—— "Geographical Studies of Rheumatoid Arthritis," P. H. Bennett and P. H. N. Wood, eds., in *Population Studies of the Rheumatic Diseases* (Amsterdam: Excerpta Medica, 1968*a*).

—— discussion in P. H. Bennett and P. H. N. Wood, eds., *Population Studies of the Rheumatic Diseases* (Amsterdam: Excerpta Medica, 1968*b*), p. 147.

—— and Jean Aitken-Swan, "Rheumatism in Miners: Part 1: Rheumatic Complaints," *British Journal of Industrial Medicine*, 9:1-18 (January 1952).

—— and John Ball, "Genetic Studies on Rheumatoid Arthritis," *Annals of the Rheumatic Diseases*, 17:160-168 (June 1958).

—— and P. H. Bennett, "Benign Polyarthritis," *Annals of the Rheumatic Diseases*, 19:20-30 (March 1960).

—— V. A. I. Laine, and Robbert de Graaff, "The Epidemiology of Rheumatoid Arthritis in Northern Europe," *Proceedings of the Royal Society of Medicine*, 54:454-462 (June 1961).

—— Robbert de Graaff, and V. A. I. Laine, "Degenerative Joint Disease in Random Samples and Occupational Groups," in M. R. Jeffrey and John Ball, eds., *The Epidemiology of Chronic Rheumatism* (Oxford: Blackwell, 1963), vol. 1, pp. 98-119.

—— J. M. Bremner, and Frieda Bier, "Osteo-arthrosis, Prevalence in the Population and Relationship between Symptoms and X-ray Changes," *Annals of the Rheumatic Diseases*, 25:1-24 (January 1966*a*).

—— —— John Ball, and T. A. Burch, "Rheumatoid Arthritis in a Subtropical Population," *Annals of the Rheumatic Diseases*, 25:59-66 (January 1966*b*).

—— T. Behrend, P. H. Bennett, J. M. Bremner, T. A. Burch, J. P. Gofton, W. O'Brien, and H. S. Robinson, "Geographical Studies on Rheumatoid Arthritis," *Annals of the Rheumatic Diseases*, 25:425-432 (September 1966*c*).

—— M. K. Molyneux, and I. Dingwall-Fordyce, "Rheumatism in Foundry Workers," *British Journal of Industrial Medicine*, 23:42-52 (January 1966*d*).

Lecocq, F. R., and J. J. McPharl, "The Effects of Starvation, High Fat Diets and Ketone Infusion on Uric Acid Balance," *Clinical Research Proceedings*, 12:274 (April 1964).

Lee, P. R., A. F. Barnett, J. F. Scholer, S. Bryner, and W. H. Clark, "Rubella Arthritis, A Study of Twenty Cases," *California Medicine*, 93:125-128 (September 1960).

Lennane, G. A. Q., B. S. Rose, and I. C. Isdale, "Gout in the Maori," *Annals of the Rheumatic Diseases*, 19:120-125 (June 1960).

le Riche, W. H., C. A. Bond, W. B. Stiver, and A. Osima, *A Linkage of Data on Physicians Services and Hospital Separations for 1960 in Ontario*, special report no. 2 (Toronto: Physicians Services Inc., 1965*a*).

—— —— —— *A Study of a Comprehensive Non-profit, Prepaid Medical Care Plan in Ontario, 1963*, special report no. 3 (Toronto: Physicians Services Inc., 1965*b*).

Lewin, T., "Osteoarthritis in Lumbar Synovial Joints: A Morphologic Study," *Acta Orthopaedica Scandinavica*, suppl. 73:1-112 (1964).

Lewis-Faning, E., "Report on an Enquiry into the Aetiologic Factors Associated with Rheumatoid Arthritis," *Annals of the Rheumatic Diseases*, suppl. to vol. 9 (1950).

—— and E. Fletcher, "A Statistical Study of 1000 Cases of Chronic Rheumatism: Part III," *Post-graduate Medical Journal*, 21:137-146 (April 1945).

Liddle, Lois, J. E. Seegmiller, and Leonard Laster, "The Enzymatic Spectrophotometric Method for Determination of Uric Acid," *Journal of Laboratory and Clinical Medicine*, 54:903-913 (December 1959).

Lieber, C. S., "Hyperuricemia Induced by Alcohol," *Arthritis and Rheumatism*, 8:786-791 (October 1965).

Lillienfeld, A. M., and B. Kordan, "A Study of Variability in the Interpretation of Chest X-rays in the Detection of Lung Cancer," *Cancer Research*, 26:2145-2147 (October 1966).

Lincoln, T. A., and Sidney Cobb, "The Prevalence of Mild Rheumatoid Arthritis in Industry," *Journal of Occupational Medicine*, 5:10-16 (January 1963).

Logan, W. P. D., and A. A. Cushion, *Morbidity Statistics from General Practice: Vol. I. General*, Studies on Medical and Population Subjects, no. 14 (London: Her Majesty's Stationer's Office, 1958).

Maclachlan, M. J., and G. P. Rodnan, "Effect of Food, Fast and Alcohol on Serum Uric Acid and Acute Attacks of Gout," *American Journal of Medicine*, 42:38-57 (January 1967).

Manheimer, R. H., K. R. C. Greene, and Frances Kroll, "Juvenile Rheumatoid Arthritis in New York City," *Archives of Pediatrics*, 76:173-185 (May 1959).

Masi, A. T., "Population Studies in Rheumatic Disease," *Annual Review of Medicine*, 18:185-206 (1967).

—— "Family, Twin, and Genetic Studies: A General Review Illustrated by Systemic Lupus Erythematosus," in P. H. Bennett and P. H. N. Wood, eds., *Population Studies of the Rheumatic Diseases* (Amsterdam: Excerpta Medica, 1968), pp. 267-286.

—— and W. A. D'Angelo, "Epidemiology of Fatal Systemic Sclerosis (Diffuse Scleroderma): A 15 Year Survey in Baltimore," *Annals of Internal Medicine*, 66:870-883 (May 1967).

—— and L. E. Shulman, "Familial Aggregation and Rheumatoid Disease," *Arthritis and Rheumatism*, 8:418-425 (June 1965).

—— Harry Robinson, and Margaret Hughen, "The Arthritis Research Program Survey of Newly Diagnosed Arthritis Among Patients of Memphis and Shelby County," *Memphis and Mid-South Medical Journal*, vol. 43, no. 11 (November 1968).

Mason, J. W., "A Review of Psychoendocrine Research on the Pituitary-adrenal Cortical System," *Psychosomatic Medicine*, 30:576-607 (September-October 1968).

Mason, R. M., R. S. Murray, J. K. Oates, and A. C. Young, "Prostatitis and Ankylosing Spondylitis," *British Medical Journal*, 1:748-751 (March 29, 1958).

May, W. P., "Rheumatoid Arthritis (Osteitis Deformans) Affecting Bones 5,500 Years Old," *British Medical Journal*, 2:1631-1632 (December 1897).

Medsger, T. A., Jr., G. P. Rodnan, John Moossy, and J. W. Vester, "Skeletal Muscle Involvement in Progressive Systemic Sclerosis," *Arthritis and Rheumatism*, 11:554-568 (August 1968).

Mendez Bryan, Ricardo, personal communication, October 15, 1963.

Merrell, Margaret, and L. E. Shulman, "Determination of the Prognosis in Chronic Disease, Illustrated by Systemic Lupus Erythematosus," *Journal of Chronic Diseases*, 1:12-32 (January 1955).

Metropolitan Life Insurance Company, "Chronic Rheumatic Diseases," *Statistical Bulletin* (May 1956), pp. 7-10.

—— "The Problem of Arthritis," *Statistical Bulletin* (February 1967), pp. 7-9.

Mikkelsen, W. M., "The Possible Association of Hyperuricemia and/or Gout with Diabetes Mellitus," *Arthritis and Rheumatism*, 8:853-859 (October 1965).

—— H. J. Dodge, I. F. Duff, F. H. Epstein, and J. A. Napier, "Clinical and Serological Estimates of the Prevalence of Rheumatoid Arthritis in the Population of Tecumseh, Michigan, 1959-1960," in M. R. Jeffrey and John Ball, eds., *The Epidemiology of Chronic Rheumatism* (Oxford: Blackwell, 1963), vol. 1, pp. 239-248.

—— —— and H. A. Valkenburg, "The Distribution of Serum Acid Levels in a

Population Unselected for Hyperuricemia or Gout," *American Journal of Medicine*, 39:242-251 (August 6, 1965).

—— —— I. F. Duff, and Hiroo Kato, "Estimates of the Prevalence of Rheumatic Diseases in the Population of Tecumseh, Michigan, 1959-60," *Journal of Chronic Diseases*, 20:351-369 (June 1967).

Ministry of Health of Great Britain, *The Incidence of Rheumatic Diseases*, Reports on Public Health and Medical Subjects, no. 23 (London: His Majesty's Stationery Office, 1924).

—— *A Report on Chronic Arthritis*, Reports on Public Health and Medical Subjects, no. 52 (London: His Majesty's Stationery Office, 1928).

Moore, C. B., and T. E. Weiss, "Uric Acid Metabolism and Myocardial Infarction," in T. N. James and J. W. Keyes, eds., *The Etiology of Myocardial Infarction* (Boston: Little, Brown & Co., 1963), pp. 459-478.

Moos, R. H., "Personality Factors Associated with Rheumatoid Arthritis: A Review," *Journal of Chronic Diseases*, 17:41-55 (January 1964).

Morris, R. D., and Sidney Cobb, unpublished.

Morteo, O. G., E. C. Franklin, Carrier McEwen, James Phython, and Martin Tanner, "Studies of Relatives of Patients with Systemic Lupus Erythematosus," *Arthritis and Rheumatism*, 4:356-363 (August 1961).

Mote, V. L., and R. L. Anderson, "An Investigation of the Effect of Misclassification on the Properties of Chi-2-tests in the Analysis of Categorical Data," *Biometrika*, 52:95-109 (June 1965).

Mott, P. E., F. C. Mann, Quin McLaughlin, and D. P. Warwick, *Shift Work: The Social, Psychological and Physical Consequences* (Ann Arbor: University of Michigan, 1965).

Murphy, Rosemary, and K. H. Shipman, "Hyperuricemia During Total Fasting," *Archives of Internal Medicine*, 112:954-959 (December 1963).

Myers, A. R., J. A. Mills, and M. W. Ropes, "The Problem of Infection in Systemic Lupus Erythematosus" (abstract), *Arthritis and Rheumatism*, 10:300 (June 1967).

Nalven, F. B., and J. F. O'Brien, "Personality Patterns of Rheumatoid Arthritic Patients," *Arthritis and Rheumatism*, 7:18-28 (February 1964).

Nasou, J. P., D. E. Kayhoe, and J. Bozicevich, "The F_{11}-Bentonite Flocculation Test for Rheumatoid Arthritis," *American Journal of Clinical Pathology*, 40:99-102 (July 1963).

National Center for Health Statistics, *Prevalence of Osteoarthritis in Adults by Age, Sex, Race and Geographic Area, United States, 1960-62*. PHS pub. no. 1000, series 11, no. 15 (Washington, D.C.: Public Health Service, June 1966a).

—— *Osteoarthritis in Adults by Selected Demographic Characteristics, 1960-1962*, PHS pub. no. 1000, series 11, no. 20 (Washington, D.C.: Public Health Service, November 1966b).

—— *Rheumatoid Arthritis in Adults, United States, 1960–1962*, PHS pub. no. 1000, series 11, no. 17 (Washington, D.C.: Public Health Service, 1966c).

—— *Osteoarthritis and Body Measurements*, PHS pub. no. 1000, series 11, no. 29 (Washington, D.C.: Public Health Service, 1968).

Nava, Pedro, and Hilton Seda, "A Ação do Pêso Corporal nos Rheumatismos," *O Hospital* (Rio de Janeiro), 66:251-263 (August 1964).

Neel, J. V., M. T. Rakic, R. T. Davidson, H. A. Valkenburg, and W. M. Mikkelsen, "Studies on Hyperuricemia: II. A Reconsideration of the Distribution of Serum Uric Acid Values in the Families of Smyth, Cotterman, and Freyberg," *American Journal of Human Genetics*, 17:14-22 (January 1965).

Nelson, S. G., and H. O. Lancaster, "A Morbidity Survey of Rheumatism in Sydney," *Medical Journal of Australia*, 46:190-193 (February 7, 1959).

Neri Serneri, G. G., and V. Bartoli, "Ricerche Genetiche sulla Predisposizione All 'artrosi' 'Dolorosa' e sui suoi Raporti con i Reumatismi Primari," *Acta Genetica Medica* (Rome), 6:503-521 (October 1957).

Nesterov, A. I., "The Clinical Course of Kashin-Beck Disease," *Arthritis and Rheumatism*, 7:29-40 (February 1964).

Neyman, J., "Outline of Statistical Treatment of the Problem of Diagnosis," *Public Health Reports* (Washington), 62:1449-1456 (October 3, 1947).

Nichols, John, A. T. Miller, Jr., and E. P. Hiatt, "Influence of Muscular Exercise on Uric Acid Excretion in Man," *Journal of Applied Physiology*, 3:501-507 (February 1951).

Nissen, H. A., and K. A. Spencer, "Psychogenic Problem (Endocrinal and Metabolic) in Chronic Arthritis," *New England Journal of Medicine*, 214:576-581 (March 19, 1936).

Nobrega, F. T., R. H. Ferguson, L. T. Kurland, and M. M. Hargraves, "Lupus Erythematosus in Rochester, Minnesota, 1950–1965: A Preliminary Study," in P. H. Bennett and P. H. N. Wood, eds., *Population Studies of the Rheumatic Diseases* (Amsterdam: Excerpta Medica, 1968), pp. 259-266.

O'Brien, W. M., "The Genetics of Rheumatoid Arthritis," *Clinical and Experimental Immunology*, 2, suppl.:785-802 (December 1967).

—— T. A. Burch, and J. J. Bunim, "Genetics of Hyperuricemia in Blackfeet and Pima Indians," *Annals of the Rheumatic Diseases*, 25:117-119 (March 1966).

—— P. H. Bennett, T. A. Burch, and J. J. Bunim, "A Genetic Study of Rheumatoid Arthritis and Rheumatoid Factor in Blackfeet and Pima Indians," *Arthritis and Rheumatism*, 10:163-179 (June 1967).

—— A. R. Clemett, and R. M. Acheson, "Symptoms and Pattern of Osteoarthritis in the Hand in the New Haven Survey of Joint Disease," in P. H. Bennett and P. H. N. Wood, eds., *Population Studies of the Rheumatic Diseases* (Amsterdam: Excerpta Medica, 1968), pp. 398-406.

Orowan, E., "The Origin of Man," *Nature*, 175:683-684 (April 16, 1955).

Oshima, Yashio, "Results of a Population Survey in Shizuoka Prefecture, July-August 1960," *Journal of Japanese Society of Internal Medicine*, 50:124-130 (1960).

—— J. Yoshimura, M. Noda, T. Kagami, I. Akaoka, and T. Nishizawa, "Gout," in *Rheumatic Diseases, Recent Advance in Japan*, Proceedings of Eighth Congress of Japanese Rheumatism Association, Okayama, 1964, p. 54.

O'Sullivan, J. B., "The Incidence of Gout and Related Uric Acid Levels in Sudbury, Massachusetts," in P. H. Bennett and P. H. N. Wood, eds., *Population Studies of the Rheumatic Diseases* (Amsterdam: Excerpta Medica, 1968), pp. 371-376.

—— E. S. Cathcart, and J. A. Bolzan, "Diagnostic Criteria and the Incidence of Rheumatoid Arthritis in Sudbury, Massachusetts," in P. H. Bennett and P. H. N. Wood, eds., *Population Studies of the Rheumatic Diseases* (Amsterdam: Excerpta Medica, 1968), pp. 109-115.

Otto, Rosemarie, and I. R. Mackay, "Psycho-social and Emotional Disturbance in Systemic Lupus Erythematosus," *Medical Journal of Australia*, 2:488-493 (September 9, 1967).

Partridge, R. E. H., J. A. D. Anderson, M. A. McCarthy, and J. J. R. Duthie, "Rheumatism in Light Industry," *Annals of the Rheumatic Diseases*, 24:332-340 (July 1965).

Perrott, G. St.J., L. M. Smith, M. Pennell, and M. E. Altenderfer, *Care of the*

Long-Term Patient: Source Book on Size and Characteristics of the Problem, PHS pub. no. 344 (Washington, D.C.: Public Health Service, 1954).

Peter, J. B., C. M. Pearson, and L. Marmor, "Erosive Osteoarthritis of the Hand," *Arthritis and Rheumatism*, 9:365-388 (June 1966).

Pilkington, T. L., "Coincidence of Rheumatoid Arthritis and Schizophrenia," *Journal of Nervous and Mental Disease*, 124:604-606 (December 1956).

Popert, A. J., and J. V. Hewitt, "Gout and Hyperuricaemia in Rural and Urban Populations," *Annals of the Rheumatic Diseases*, 21:154-163 (June 1962).

Praetorius, E., "An Enzymatic Method for the Determination of Uric Acid by Ultraviolet Spectrophotometry," *Scandinavian Journal of Clinical and Laboratory Investigation*, 1:222-230 (1949).

—— and H. E. Poulsen, "Enzymatic Determination of Uric Acid with Detailed Directions," *Scandinavian Journal of Clinical and Laboratory Investigation*, 5:273-280 (1953).

Price, G. E., D. K. Ford, J. P. Gofton, and H. S. Robinson, "An Outbreak of 'Infectious' Polyarthritis in a Haida Indiana Family," *Arthritis and Rheumatism*, 6:633-638 (October 1963).

Prick, J. J. G., and K. J. M. van de Loo, *The Psychosomatic Approach to Primary Chronic Rheumatoid Arthritis*, T. G. Faly, trans. (Philadelphia: Davis, 1964).

Prior, I. A. M., B. S. Rose, H. P. B. Harvey, and F. Davidson, "Hyperuricemia, Gout and Diabetic Abnormality in Polynesian People," *Lancet*, 1:333-338 (February 12, 1966).

Rahe, R. H., and R. J. Arthur, "Stressful Underwater Demolition Training: Serum Urate and Cholesterol Variability," *Journal of the American Medical Association*, 202:1052-1054 (December 11, 1967).

—— R. T. Rubin, R. J. Arthur, and B. R. Clark, "Serum Uric Acid and Cholesterol Variability, A Comprehensive View of Underwater Demolition Team Training," *Journal of the American Medical Association*, 206:2875-2880 (December 23-30, 1968).

Rakic, M. T., H. A. Valkenburg, R. T. Davidson, J. P. Engels, W. M. Mikkelsen, J. V. Neel, and I. F. Duff, with D. S. Himes, "Observations on the Natural History of Hyperuricemia and Gout: I. An Eighteen Year Follow-up of Nineteen Gouty Families," *American Journal of Medicine*, 37:862-871 (December 1964).

Reynolds, W. E., "Report from the Subcommittee on Diagnostic Criteria for Systemic Lupus Erythematosus," in P. H. Bennett and P. H. N. Wood, eds., *Population Studies of the Rheumatic Diseases* (Amsterdam: Excerpta Medica, 1968), pp. 287-289.

—— personal communication, April 30, 1969.

Rich, A. R., "The Role of Hypersensitivity in Periarteritis Nodosa: As Indicated by Seven Cases Developing during Serum Sickness and Sulfonamide Therapy," *Bulletin of the Johns Hopkins Hospital*, 71:123-140 (September 1942).

Rimoin, D. L., and J. E. Wennberg, "Acute Septic Arthritis Complicating Chronic Rheumatoid Arthritis," *Journal of the American Medical Association*, 196: 617-621 (May 16, 1966).

Rimón, Ranan, "A Psychosomatic Approach to Rheumatoid Arthritis: A Clinical Study of 100 Female Patients," *Acta Rheumatologica Scandinavica*, suppl. no. 13 (1969).

Rinehart, R. E., and Helen Marcus, "Incidence of Amebiasis in Healthy Individuals, Clinic Patients and Those with Rheumatoid Arthritis," *Northwest Medicine*, 54:708-712 (July 1955).

Robecchi, A., " 'Poliartrosi' e 'Artrosi primitiva' alla Luce delle Osservatione Cliniche," *Minerva Medica*, 55:2157-2161 (July 7, 1964).

Rodnan, G. P., "The Natural History of Progressive Systemic Sclerosis (Diffuse Scleroderma)," *Bulletin on the Rheumatic Diseases*, 13:301-304 (February 1963).

Roemmich, William, "Disability and Rheumatic Diseases: Social Security Data," *Archives of Environmental Health* (Chicago), 4:490-491 (May 1962).

Romanus, Ragnar, "Pelvo-spondylitis Ossificans in the Male and Genitourinary Infection," *Acta Medica Scandinavica* suppl. 280 (1953).

Ropes, M. W., and Walter Bauer, *Synovial Fluid Changes in Joint Diseases* (Cambridge, Mass.: Harvard University Press, 1953).

—— G. A. Bennett, Sidney Cobb, R. F. Jacox, and R. A. Jessar, "Proposed Diagnostic Criteria for Rheumatoid Arthritis," *Annals of the Rheumatic Diseases*, 16:118-125 (March 1957).

—— —— —— —— —— "1958 Revision of Diagnostic Criteria for Rheumatoid Arthritis," *Arthritis and Rheumatism*, 2:16-20 (February 1959).

Rose, B. S., I. A. M. Prior, and F. Davidson, "Gout and Hyperuricaemia in New Zealand and Polynesia," in P. H. Bennett and P. H. N. Wood, eds., *Population Studies of the Rheumatic Diseases* (Amsterdam: Excerpta Medica, 1968), pp. 344-353.

Rothermich, N. O., and V. K. Philips, "Rheumatoid Arthritis in Criminal and Mentally Ill Populations," *Arthritis and Rheumatism*, 6:639–640 (October 1963).

Rubin, Theodore, Joseph Rosenbaum, and Sidney Cobb, "The Use of Interview Data for the Detection of Associations in Field Studies," *Journal of Chronic Diseases*, 4:253-266 (September 1956).

Ruffer, M. A., *Studies in the Paleopathology of Egypt* (Chicago: University of Chicago Press, 1921).

Sappington, C. O., "A Study of the Morbidity and Accident Experience of a Boston Public Utility During the Period 1918-22," unpublished dissertation, Harvard School of Public Health, 1924.

Saskatchewan Department of Public Health, *Statistical Tables Supplementing the Annual Reports of the Saskatchewan Hospital Services Plan, 1965 and the Saskatchewan Medical Care Insurance Commission, 1965*, Regina (Saskatchewan), 1966.

Saville, P. D., "A Quantitative Approach to Simple Radiographic Diagnosis of Osteoporosis: Its Application to the Osteoporosis of Rheumatoid Arthritis," *Arthritis and Rheumatism*, 10:416-422 (October 1967).

Schmid, F. R., and H. Slatis, "Clinical and Serological Abnormalities in the Families of Patients with Rheumatoid Arthritis," in *Atti del X Congresso della Lega Internazionale contro il Rheumatismo* (Turin: Minerva Medica, 1961), vol. 2, p. 739.

Schnitker, M. A., "A History of the Treatment of Gout," *Bulletin of the History of Medicine*, 4:89-120 (February 1936).

Schubart, A. F., A. S. Cohen, and Evan Calkins, "Latex Fixation Test in Rheumatoid Arthritis: III. A Longitudinal Study of the Titer of Rheumatoid Factor and Thermolabile Inhibitor," *Arthritis and Rheumatism*, 7:8-17 (February 1964).

Schull, W. J., and Sidney Cobb, "Intrafamilial Transmission of Rheumatoid Arthritis: III. The Lack of Support for a Genetic Hypothesis," *Journal of Chronic Diseases*, 22:217-222 (September 1969).

Scott, J. T., F. M. McCollum, and V. P. Holloway, "Starvation, Ketosis, and Uric

Acid Excretion" (abstract), *Annals of the Rheumatic Diseases*, 23:83 (January 1964).

Seegmiller, J. E., R. R. Howell, and S. E. Malawista, "The Inflammatory Reaction to Sodium Urate: Its Possible Relationship to the Genesis of Acute Gouty Arthritis," *Journal of the American Medical Association*, 180:469-475 (May 12, 1962).

Sever, E. D., "Extra-articular Manifestations of Rheumatoid Arthritis," *British Journal of Clinical Practice*, 19:637-644 (November 1965).

Shapiro, J. R., J. R. Klinenberg, William Peck, S. E. Goldfinger, and J. E. Seegmiller, "Hyperuricemia Associated with Obesity and Intensified by Caloric Restrictions" (abstract), *Arthritis and Rheumatism*, 7:343 (June 1964).

Sherwood, K. K., personal communication to Dr. Joseph Zubin, January 10, 1963.

Shichikawa, Kanji, and Y. Komatsubara, "La Goutte au Japon," *Revue du Rhumatisme et des Maladies Osteo-Articulaires*, 31:13-16 (January-February 1964).

—— A. Mayeda, Y. Komatsubara, T. Yamamoto, O. Akabori, I. Hongo, T. Kosugi, T. Miyauchi, M. Orihasa, and A. Taniguchi, "Rheumatic Complaints in Urban and Rural Populations in Osaka," *Annals of the Rheumatic Diseases*, 25:25-31 (January 1966).

Short, C. L., Walter Bauer, and W. E. Reynolds, *Rheumatoid Arthritis* (Cambridge, Mass.: Harvard University Press, 1957).

Siegel, Morris, and S. L. Lee, "The Epidemiology of Systemic Lupus Erythematosus: Results of a Population Study in New York City," in P. H. Bennett and P. H. N. Wood, eds., *Population Studies of the Rheumatic Diseases* (Amsterdam: Excerpta Medica, 1968), pp. 245-258.

—— —— D. Widelock, N. V. Gwon, and H. Kravitz, "A Comparative Family Study of Rheumatoid Arthritis and Systemic Lupus Erythematosus," *New England Journal of Medicine*, 273:893-897 (October 21, 1965).

—— —— and N. S. Peress, "The Epidemiology of Drug-Induced Systemic Lupus Erythematosus," *Arthritis and Rheumatism*, 10:407-414 (October 1967).

Sitaj, Stephan, and M. Šebo, "Rheumatoid Arthritis and Ankylosing Spondylitis in Czechoslovakia," in P. H. Bennett and P. H. N. Wood, eds., *Population Studies of the Rheumatic Diseases* (Amsterdam: Excerpta Medica, 1968), pp. 64-66.

—— L. Straka, and G. Niepel, "The Occurrence of Rheumatic Diseases on the Basis of an Examination of the Population as a Whole," *Bratislavské Lekarske Listy*, 34:612-639 (June 1954).

—— V. Svec, and T. Urbanek, "K Otazke Tzv. Epizodickych Benigych Artritid," *Vnitrni Lekarstvi*, 10:565-574 (1964).

Smyth, C. J., "Hereditary Factors in Gout: A Review of Recent Literature," *Metabolism: Clinical and Experimental*, 6:218-229 (May 1957).

—— C. W. Cotterman, and R. H. Freyberg, "The Genetics of Gout and Hyperuricemia: An Analysis of Nineteen Families," *Journal of Clinical Investigation*, 27:749-759 (November 1948).

Sokoloff, Leon, "The Biology of Degenerative Joint Disease," *Perspectives in Biology and Medicine*, 7:94-106 (autumn 1963).

Solomon, G. F., and R. H. Moos, "Emotions, Immunity, and Disease," *Archives of General Psychiatry*, 11:657-674 (December 1964).

Spiegel, R., "Clinical Aspects of Periarteritis Nodosa," *Archives of Internal Medicine*, 58:993-1040 (December 1936).

Stecher, R. M., "Heberden's Nodes: The Incidence of Hypertrophic Arthritis of the Fingers," *New England Journal of Medicine*, 222:300-308 (February 22, 1940).

—— "Heberden's Nodes: A Clinical Description of Osteoarthritis of the Finger Joints (Heberden Oration)," *Annals of the Rheumatic Diseases*, 14:1-10 (March 1955).

—— *Documenta Rheumatologica: Heredity in Joint Diseases* (Basel: Geigy, 1957).

Stecher, R. M., A. H. Hersh, and W. M. Solomon, "The Heredity of Gout and Its Relationship to Familial Hyperuricemia," *Annals of Internal Medicine*, 31: 595-614 (October 1949).

Steinbrocker, O., C. H. Traeger, and R. C. Batterman, "Therapeutic Criteria in Rheumatoid Arthritis," *Journal of the American Medical Association*, 140: 659-662 (June 25, 1949).

Steiner, F. J. F., F. Westendorp-Boerma, J. J. de Blécourt, and H. A. Valkenburg, "Prevalence of Rheumatic Diseases on the Coastal Island of Marken," in P. H. Bennett and P. H. N. Wood, eds., *Population Studies of the Rheumatic Diseases* (Amsterdam: Excerpta Medica, 1968), pp. 67-69.

Stetten, DeWitt, Jr., and J. Z. Hearon, "Intellectual Level Measured by Army Classification Battery and Serum Uric Acid Concentration," *Science*, 129: 1737 (June 26, 1959).

Steuermann, Nicholas, and A. H. Farias, "Hyperuricemia in Filipinos," *Hawaii Medical Journal*, 20:151-153 (November-December 1960).

Steven, G. D., " 'Standard Bone': A Description of Radiographic Technique," *Annals of the Rheumatic Diseases*, 6:184-185 (September 1947).

Stocks, Percy, "Survey of Sickness Prevalence: March Quarter, 1948," *Monthly Bulletin of the Ministry of Health and the Public Health Laboratory Service*, Great Britain, 7:213–219 (October 1948).

Survey Research Center, *Interviewers' Manual* (Ann Arbor, Mich.: Institute for Social Research, March 1966).

Sury, Børge, *Rheumatoid Arthritis in Children: A Clinical Study* (Copenhagen: Munksgaard, 1952).

Svanborg, Alvar, and Lennart Sölvell, "Incidence of Disseminated Lupus Erythematosus," *Journal of the American Medical Association*, 1965:1126-1128 (November 2, 1957).

Svec, K. H., and J. H. Dingle, "The Occurrence of Rheumatoid Factor in Association with Antibody Response to Influenza A2 (Asian) Virus," *Arthritis and Rheumatism*, 8:524-539 (August 1965).

Sydenham, Thomas, *Observationes Medicae circa Morbum Acutoram Historiam et Curiationem* (London: G. Kettilby, 1676, as trans. by R. G. Latham, *The Works of Thomas Sydenham* (London: Sydenham Society, 1848), vol. 1.

—— *Tractatus de Podagra et Hydrope* (London: G. Kettilby, 1783, as trans. by R. G. Latham, *The Works of Thomas Sydenham* (London: Sydenham Society, 1848), vol. 2.

Talbott, J. H., "Serum Urate in Relatives of Gouty Patients," *Journal of Clinical Investigation*, 19:645-648 (July 1940).

—— *Gout*, 2nd ed. (New York: Grune and Stratton, 1964).

Tegner, W. S., "Social Aspects of the Rheumatic Diseases," in W. S. C. Copeman, ed., *Textbook of the Rheumatic Diseases* (Edinburgh: Livingston, 1964).

Tempelaar, H. C. G., and J. van Breemen, "Communication of the Consulting Bureau at Amsterdam: Rheumatism and Occupation," *Acta Rheumatologica*, 4:36-38 (August-September 1932).

Trevathan, R. D., and J. C. Tatum, "Rarity of Concurrence of Psychosis and Rheumatoid Arthritis in Individual Patients," *Journal of Nervous and Mental Diseases*, 120:83-84 (July-August 1954).

Trowell, H. C., *Non-Infective Disease in Africa* (London: Arnold, 1960).

U.S. Bureau of the Census, *Mortality Statistics 1936* (Washington, D.C.: Department of Commerce, 1938).

U.S. Department of Health, Education, and Welfare, *Occupational Characteristics of Disabled Workers, by Disabling Condition: Disability Insurance Benefit Awards Made in 1959-1962 to Men under Age 65*, PHS pub. no. 1531 (Washington, D.C.: Public Health Service, 1967).

U.S. National Health Survey, *The Hawaii Health Survey: Description and Selected Results, Oahu, Hawaii, October 1958-September 1959*, PHS pub. no. 584-C3 (Washington, D.C.: Public Health Service, May 1960a).

—— *Arthritis and Rheumatism Reported in Interviews, United States, July 1957-June 1959*, PHS pub. no. 584-B20 (Washington, D.C.: Public Health Service, September 1960b).

U.S. Public Health Service, *Arthritis Source Book*, PHS pub. no. 1431 (Washington, D.C.: Public Health Service, April 1966).

See also National Center for Health Statistics.

Valkenburg, H. A., "Rheumatoid Factor Tests," *Milbank Memorial Fund Quarterly*, 43:153-160 (April 1965).

—— "Observer Variance and Prevalence of Rheumatoid Arthritis and Osteoarthritis in a Longitudinal Population Study in the Netherlands," in P. H. Bennett and P. H. N. Wood, eds., *Population Studies of the Rheumatic Diseases* (Amsterdam: Excerpta Medica, 1968), pp. 93-98.

—— John Ball, T. A. Burch, P. H. Bennett, and J. S. Lawrence, "Rheumatoid Factors in a Rural Population," *Annals of the Rheumatic Diseases*, 25:497-508 (November 1966).

van Dam, G., A. Lezwign, and J. G. Bos, "Death-rate of Patients with Rheumatoid Arthritis," *Atti del X Congresso della Lega Internazionale contro il Rheumatismo* (Turin: Minerva Medica, 1961), vol. 1, p. 161.

Waine, Hans, Dagmar Nevinny, Joseph Rosenthal, and I. B. Joffe, "Association of Osteoarthritis and Diabetes Mellitus," *Tufts Folia Medica — Bulletin of the Tufts-New England Medical Center*, 7:13-19 (January-March 1961).

Wardle, E. N., "Primary Generalized Chronic Arthritis," *Rheumatism* (London), 9:51-57 (July 1953).

Weiss, R. J., and B. J. Bergen, "Social Supports and the Reduction of Psychiatric Disability," *Psychiatry*, 31:107-115 (May 1968).

Whittinghill, M., E. E. Hendricks, G. S. Taylor, and L. S. Thorp, "The Distribution of Rheumatoid Arthritis, Spondylitis and Still's Disease in a Single Large Kindred," in *Proceedings of the Tenth International Congress on Genetics* (Toronto: University of Toronto Press, 1959), vol. 2, p. 314.

Wilson, Donald, "The Familial History of Gout," *Proceedings of the Royal Society of Medicine*, 44:285-288 (April 1951).

Wood, J. W., Hiroo Kato, K. G. Johnson, Yutaka Uda, W. J. Russell, and I. F. Duff, "Rheumatoid Arthritis in Hiroshima and Nagasaki, Japan: Prevalence, Incidence and Clinical Characteristics," *Arthritis and Rheumatism*, 10:21-31 (February 1967).

Wood, P. H. N., "Age and the Rheumatic Diseases," in P. H. Bennett and P. H. N. Wood, eds., *Population Studies of the Rheumatic Diseases* (Amsterdam: Excerpta Medica, 1968), pp. 26-38.

Woolsey, T. D., "Prevalence of Arthritis and Rheumatism in the United States," *Public Health Reports*, 67:505-512 (June 1952).

Wright, V., and G. Watkinson, "Sacro-iliitis and ulcerative colitis," *British Medical Journal*, 2:675-679 (September 18, 1965).

Wyatt, B. L., *Chronic Arthritis and Fibrositis* (Baltimore, Md.: William Wood, 1933).

Youden, W. J., "Index for Rating Diagnostic Tests," *Cancer*, 3:32-35 (January 1950).

Yu, T'sai-Fan, J. H. Sirota, L. Berger, M. Halpern, and A. B. Gutman, "Effect of Sodium Lactate Infusion on Urate Clearance in Man," *Proceedings of the Society for Experimental Biology and Medicine*, 96:809-813 (December 1957).

Zachau-Christiansen, B., "The Rise in the Serum Uric Acid during Muscular Exercise," *Scandinavian Journal of Clinical and Laboratory Investigation*, 11:57-60 (1959).

Zborowski, Mark, "Cultural Components in Response to Pain," *Journal of Social Issues*, 8, no. 4, 16-30 (1952).

Ziff, Morris, F. R. Schmid, A. J. Lewis, Martin Tanner, "Familial Occurrence of the Rheumatoid Factor," *Arthritis and Rheumatism*, 1:392-399 (October 1958).

INDEX

Age distribution
  ankylosing spondylitis, 107, 108
  cohort effects, 43
  dermatomyositis, 98, 99
  disk degeneration, 70
  gout, 85
  juvenile rheumatoid arthritis, 110, 111, 112
  lupus erythematosus, 98-103 *passim*
  osteoarthrosis, 67-69, 71, 72, 77, 79
  polyarteritis nodosa, 98, 99
  rheumatic complaints, 14-15, 16
  rheumatic disease disability, 8, 9
  rheumatoid disease, 33, 35, 39, 40, 42-44, 45, 46, 98, 99
  scleroderma, 98, 99
  uric acid levels, 90
Ankylosing spondylitis, 105-114
  relation to rheumatoid disease, 106
Association with other diseases. *See* Disease association

Bias in self-report, 4. *See also* Observer variation

Collagen disease. *See* Connective-tissue disorders
Connective-tissue disorders, 62, 97-104, 113
  interrelationship among, 53, 97
Criteria, diagnostic. *See* Diagnostic criteria

Degenerative joint disease, 63-80
Depression
  juvenile rheumatoid arthritis, 113
  rheumatoid disease, 57, 60
Dermatomyositis, 97, 99, 100, 102
Diagnostic criteria
  ankylosing spondylitis, 105-107
  basic principles, 2, 3, 18
  disk degeneration, 63, 77
  gout, 81-82
  juvenile rheumatoid arthritis, 110-111
  lupus erythematosus, 103, 104
  osteoarthrosis, 63-64, 77
  rheumatoid disease, 19-28, 36, 37, 97
Disability
  ankylosing spondylitis, 116
  disk degeneration, 79, 80, 115, 116, 118
  gout, 118
  osteoarthrosis, 79, 80, 116, 118
  rheumatic diseases, 7-9
  rheumatoid disease, 15, 16, 39, 115-118, 119
Disease association
  ankylosing spondylitis, 97, 108-109
  connective-tissue disorders, 104

dermatomyositis, 97
  gout, 118
  juvenile rheumatoid arthritis, 113
  lupus erythematosus, 53, 97, 103
  osteoarthrosis, 71, 75, 79, 118
  polyarteritis nodosa, 53, 97
  rheumatoid disease, 40, 52-55, 60-61, 97, 118
  scleroderma, 53, 97
Disk degeneration, 63-80
  association with osteoarthrosis, 65, 77

Etiology
  lupus erythematosus, 103
  osteoarthrosis, 65, 70-71
  polyarteritis nodosa, 101-102
  rheumatic diseases, 4-5
  rheumatoid disease, 61-62, 118

Family structure in rheumatoid disease, 49-50, 56, 57-58

Genetics
  ankylosing spondylitis, 109-110
  connective-tissue disorders, 62, 103, 119
  gout, 52, 94-95
  juvenile rheumatoid arthritis, 112-113
  lupus erythematosus, 103
  osteoarthrosis, 76-78, 79
  rheumatoid disease, 51-52, 62
  uric acid level, 96
Geographic distribution
  ankylosing spondylitis, 107-108
  dermatomyositis, 98, 100, 101
  disk degeneration, 70
  gout, 82-84, 87, 96
  lupus erythematosus, 98, 100, 101
  osteoarthrosis, 67-69, 79
  polyarteritis nodosa, 98, 100
  rheumatic complaints, 12-14
  rheumatoid disease, 29, 45-48, 98, 100, 101
  scleroderma, 98, 100
  uric acid levels, 88-89, 96
Gout, 52, 81-96, 118
  colchicine response, 81
  See also Uric acid

Heberden's nodes. *See* Osteophytes
Historical references
  gout, 82
  rheumatic diseases, 5
  rheumatoid disease, 18-19, 44-45
Hostility
  juvenile rheumatoid arthritis, 113
  rheumatoid disease, 49, 57-60, 62

Hyperuricemia, 81-96

Incidence
  gout, 84
  juvenile rheumatoid arthritis, 111-112
  rheumatic diseases, 8
  rheumatoid disease, 29-30
Infection
  juvenile rheumatoid arthritis, 111, 113,
    114
  lupus erythematosus, 103
  polyarteritis nodosa, 101-102
  rheumatoid disease, 53-55, 61, 62

Juvenile rheumatoid arthritis, 105-114

Longitudinal studies
  osteoarthrosis, 80
  rheumatoid disease, 30-37, 119
Lupus erythematosus, 52, 53, 97, 99, 100,
  102-103

Marital status
  dermatomyositis, 100
  lupus erythematosus, 100
  polyarteritis nodosa, 100
  rheumatoid disease, 50, 56, 100
  scleroderma, 100
Medical care
  adequacy of, 36-38, 115-119
  ankylosing spondylitis, 117
  disk degeneration, 80
  frequency of, 36-38, 40, 115-119
  gout, 96, 117
  nonmedical, 10
  osteoarthrosis, 80, 117
  rheumatic diseases, 9-11
  rheumatoid disease, 49, 117, 119
Mortality
  dermatomyositis, 98-101, 102
  juvenile rheumatoid arthritis, 99, 111
  lupus erythematosus, 97-101, 102
  osteoarthrosis, 78
  polyarteritis nodosa, 98-101
  rheumatic diseases, 6, 7
  rheumatoid disease, 29, 38-41, 49, 98-101
  scleroderma, 98-101, 102

Obesity
  disk degeneration, 73
  osteoarthrosis, 71, 73-74, 77, 79
  uric acid level, 91, 92
Observer variation
  ankylosing spondylitis, 106-107
  disk degeneration, 67
  osteoarthrosis, 66-67
  rheumatoid disease, 20-25, 27, 34-36
  See also Bias in self-report

Occupation
  disk degeneration, 75, 76
  gout, 92-93, 96
  osteoarthrosis, 71, 74-76
  rheumatoid disease, 15-16, 51
  scleroderma, 102
Osteoarthrosis, 63-80
  association with disk degeneration, 65
  interfacetal joints of spine, 65
  primary, 64-65, 77
  progression, 71, 72, 77
  secondary, 65, 77
  wear-and-tear theory, 75
Osteophytes, 63, 64, 65, 77, 78
Osteoporosis, 22

Pain
  ankylosing spondylitis, 105
  disk degeneration, 64, 78-79
  gout, 81
  osteoarthrosis, 63-64, 78-79
  rheumatoid disease, 33-37 passim
Pain in joints, 4
Personality in rheumatoid disease, 57, 62
Podagra, 81
Poliomyelitic paralysis, 71, 75
Polyarteritis nodosa, 53, 97, 99, 100,
  101-102
Prevalence
  ankylosing spondylitis, 107-108, 114
  disk degeneration, 69-70
  gout, 82-84, 85-86, 93, 94, 96
  juvenile rheumatoid arthritis, 111-112, 114
  lupus erythematosus, 102
  osteoarthrosis, 67-69
  renal stone, 86, 87, 96
  rheumatic complaints, 6, 11-14
  rheumatoid disease, 28-29, 34, 41, 42-44,
    45-50 passim
Progressive systemic sclerosis. See
  Scleroderma
Protep, 4, 30-36, 51
Psychological factors
  juvenile rheumatoid arthritis, 113
  rheumatoid disease, 56-62

Race
  dermatomyositis, 98, 100, 101
  gout, 83, 85, 94
  lupus erythematosus, 98, 100, 101, 103
  osteoarthrosis, 68
  polyarteritis nodosa, 98, 100
  rheumatoid disease, 48-49, 50, 56, 98, 100
  scleroderma, 98, 100, 101
  uric acid levels, 89
Renal stone, 86, 87, 90, 96
Rheumatic complaints, 6-16, 115-119
Rheumatic diseases, basic concepts, 1-5

Rheumatic fever, 52, 53, 113
Rheumatoid arthritis, *See* Rheumatoid
  disease
Rheumatoid disease
  clinical polyarthritis, 42
  epidemiology of, 42-62
  frequency of, 17-41
  mortality, 38-41, 49, 98-101
  progression, 30-36
  remittancy, 30-31
Rheumatoid factors. *See* Serological tests
Rheumatoid spondylitis. *See* Ankylosing
  spondylitis

Sacroiliitis
  ankylosing spondylitis, 105-106, 108
  juvenile rheumatoid arthritis, 112
Scleroderma, 97, 99, 100, 102
Seasonal variation in rheumatoid arthritis, 51
Serological tests, 23, 24-25, 27-28
Serum uric acid. *See* Uric acid
Severity gradient, 2, 3
  disk degeneration, 69, 70
  gout, 118
  osteoarthrosis, 68-69, 118
  rheumatic complaints, 14-16
  rheumatic diseases, 6, 7, 8
  rheumatoid disease, 2, 17, 18-19, 31, 33,
    118
Sex distribution
  dermatomyositis, 98-101 *passim*
  disk degeneration, 69-70
  gout, 83-86 *passim,* 94
  juvenile rheumatoid arthritis, 110, 111,
    112
  lupus erythematosus, 98-103 *passim*
  osteoarthrosis, 65, 68-74 *passim,* 78
  polyarteritis nodosa, 98, 99, 100
  rheumatic complaints, 14, 16
  rheumatic diseases, 8, 9, 115-118
  rheumatoid disease, 29, 39-53 *passim,*
    57-60, 98, 99, 100
  scleroderma, 98-101 *passim*
  uric acid level, 88, 89, 90-91
Sick absences. *See* Disability
Sjøgren's syndrome, 52, 53, 113
Social environment
  gout, 92-93
  juvenile rheumatoid arthritis, 113-114
  osteoarthrosis, 78
  rheumatoid disease, 49, 50, 57-58, 61-62

uric acid level, 92, 96
Socioeconomic distribution
  disk degeneration, 75, 76
  gout, 85, 92
  osteoarthrosis, 74-78 *passim*
  rheumatic complaints, 15-16
  rheumatoid disease, 49, 51, 56
Status stress in rheumatoid disease, 56,
  57-58
Still's disease. *See* Juvenile rheumatoid
  arthritis
Surveys, interview
  rheumatic complaints, 11-13
  rheumatic diseases, 9
  rheumatoid disease, 23, 26-27
Surveys, medical
  gout, 82-84, 85-87, 94-95
  juvenile rheumatoid arthritis, 111
  osteoarthrosis, 78-80
  rheumatic complaints, 11-14
  rheumatic diseases, 5, 7
  uric acid level, 87-90
Systemic lupus erythematosus. *See* Lupus
  erythematosus

Tophi, 81
Trauma
  juvenile rheumatoid arthritis, 113, 114
  osteoarthrosis, 65
  rheumatoid disease, 55, 61, 62

Uric acid
  biochemical tests for, 85, 87-89, 95-96
  crystals, 81, 93
  diet, 92
  drugs, 92
  factors influencing level, 90-93
  and gout, 81, 82
  hyperuricemia, 85, 89-90, 95
  social status, 92, 93
  and various diseases, 91, 93

Wear-and-tear theory for osteoarthrosis,
  71-78, 118

X-ray, 1
  ankylosing spondylitis, 105-106, 107, 108,
    114
  disk degeneration, 69-70
  osteoarthrosis, 63, 64, 66-69
  rheumatoid disease, 22-24, 27-28